DRUG NAMES AND CLASSIFICATIONS

How to use this book

This book, which consists entirely of drug names and classifications, has over 1,000 entries—all arranged alphabetically by generic drug name.

Information is arranged in a convenient two-column format. The left column lists the generic drug name, alternate generics in parentheses (if applicable), and the therapeutic and pharmacologic classifications. The right column lists trade names in alphabetical order. Combination products are marked with an asterisk (*). Products available in Canada only are marked with a dagger (†); those available in Australia only are marked with a double dagger (‡). For example:

aminophylline (theophylline ethylenediamine) T: bronchodilator P: xanthine derivative	Aminophyllin, Amodrine*, Amphedrine Compound*, Asmadrin*, Asminorel*, B.M.E.*, Bronchovent*, Cardophyllin‡, Corophyllin†, Mudrane GG-2*, Neogen*, Phyllocontin, Romaphed*, Somophyllin-DF, Strema*

The index contains all trade names and classifications.

A

GENERIC NAME AND CLASSIFICATIONS	TRADE NAMES
acebutolol T: antihypertensive, antiarrhythmic P: beta-adrenergic blocking agent	Monitan†, Sectral
acetaminophen (paracetamol) T: nonnarcotic analgesic, antipyretic P: para-aminophenol derivative	Acephen, Aceta, Ace-Tabs†, Acetaminophen Uniserts, Aceta with Codeine*, Actamin, Actamin Extra, Akes-n-Pain*, Allerest*, Allerest Sinus Pain Formula*, Alumadrine*, Amaphen*, Amino-Bar*, Aminodyne*, Anacin-3, Anacin-3 Maximum Strength, Anodynos Forte*, Anuphen, Apacet, Apacet Extra Strength, Apacet Oral Solution, APAP, Apo-Acetaminophen†, Arthragen*, Atasol†, Atasol Forte†, Bancaps*, Banesin, Blanex*, Bowman Cold*, BQ Cold*, Bromo Seltzer*, Campain†, Ceetamol‡, Chexit*, Children's Anacin-3, Children's Apacet, Children's Genapap, Children's Panadol, Children's Tylenol, Children's Ty-Pap, Children's Ty-Tabs, Codalan*, Codimal*, Colrex Compound*, Comtrex*, Conar*, Conar-A*, Conex*, Congesprin*, Contac*, Coricidin Sinus Headache*, Co-Tylenol*, Dapa, Darvocet-N*, Darvocet-N 100*, Datril, Datril Extra Strength, Demerol APAP*, Dengesic*, Dolanex, Dolar Plus*, Dolene AP-65*, Drinophen*, Dularin-TH*, Duoprin*, Dymadon‡, Emagrin Forte*, Esgic*, Excedrin*, Exdol†, Exdol Strong†, F.C.A.H.*, Fendol*, Gaysal-S*, Genapap, Genebs, Genebs Extra Strength, Gentabs, Halenol, Histogesic*, Histosal #2*, Hycomine Compound*, Hydrocet*, Infant's Anacin-3, Infant's Apacet, Infant's Tylenol, Infant's Ty-Pap, Junior Disprol‡, Kiddies Sialco*, Kleer*, Koly-Tabs*, Koryza*, Liquiprin, Meda Cap, MedaTab, *(continued)*

GENERIC NAME AND CLASSIFICATIONS	TRADE NAMES
acetaminophen *(continued)*	Midrin*, Minotal*, Myapap, Myocalm*, N-D Gesic*, Neopap, Nyquil*, Oraphen-PD, Ornex*, Pamprin*, Panadol, Panadol Junior Strength, Panamax‡, Panex, Panitol*, Panritis*, Parafon Forte*, Paraphen†, Parmol‡, Partuss-A*, Pedric, Percocet-5*, Percogesic*, Phenaphen, Phenaphen #2*, Phenaphen #3*, Phenaphen #4*, Phenaphen-650*, Phrenilin*, Phrenilin Forte*, Phrenilin with Codeine*, Presalin*, Proval #3*, Renpap*, Rentuss*, Repan*, Rhinex*, Rhinogesic*, Robigesic†, Rounox†, S.A.C. Sinus*, Saleto*, Saleto-D*, Salocol*, Salphenyl*, Santussin*, Scotgesic*, Scotuss*, Sedacane*, Sedalgesic*, Sedragesic*, Sialco*, Sinarest*, Sine-Aid*, Sine-Off*, Sinubid*, Sinulin*, Sinus Tab*, Sinutab*, Spantuss*, Statomin Maleate II*, Super-Anahist*, Suppap, Talacen*, Tapanol, Tapanol Extra Strength, Tempra, Tenol, Triaminicin*, Triapin*, Tussagesic*, Two-Dyne*, Ty Caplets, Ty Caps, Tylenol, Tylenol Extra Strength, Tylenol with Codeine*, Tylox*, Ty Tabs, Valadol, Valihist*, Valorin, Vicks Children's Cough Syrup*, Vicks Daycare*, Wygesic*
acetazolamide T: adjunctive treatment for open-angle glaucoma and perioperative treatment for acute angle-closure glaucoma, anticonvulsant, management of edema, prevention and treatment of acute high-altitude sickness P: carbonic anhydrase inhibitor	Acetazolam†, Ak-Zol, Apo-Acetazolamide†, Dazamide, Diamox, Diamox Sequels, Storzolamide

T Therapeutic classification.   P Pharmacologic classification.

GENERIC NAME AND CLASSIFICATIONS	TRADE NAMES
acetazolamide sodium T: adjunctive treatment for open-angle glaucoma and perioperative treatment for acute angle-closure glaucoma, anticonvulsant, management of edema, prevention and treatment of acute high-altitude sickness P: carbonic anhydrase inhibitor	Diamox Parenteral, Diamox Sodium†
acetic acid T: antibacterial, antifungal P: acid	Coly-Mycin-S Otic*, Domeboro Otic, Otocalm-H Ear Drops*, Otostan HC*, VōSol Otic Solution
acetohexamide T: antidiabetic agent P: sulfonylurea	Dimelor†, Dymelor
acetohydroxamic acid T: antiurolithic, adjunctive agent in treatment of urinary tract infection P: urease inhibitor	Lithostat
acetophenazine maleate T: antipsychotic P: phenothiazine (piperazine derivative)	Tindal
acetylcholine chloride T: miotic P: cholinergic agonist	Miochol
acetylcysteine T: mucolytic agent, antidote for acetaminophen overdose P: amino acid (L-cysteine) derivative	Airbron†, Mucomyst, Mucosol, Parvolex‡
activated charcoal T: antidote, antidiarrheal, antiflatuent P: adsorbent	Actidose-Aqua, Charcoaide, Charcocaps, Liqui-Char, Superchar
acyclovir (acycloguanosine) T: antiviral agent P: synthetic purine nucleoside	Zovirax
acyclovir sodium T: antiviral agent P: synthetic purine nucleoside	Zovirax

---

† Available in Canada only.   ‡ Available in Australia only.   * Combination product.

GENERIC NAME AND CLASSIFICATIONS	TRADE NAMES
adenosine T: antiarrhythmic P: nucleoside	Adenocard
albumin 5% T: plasma volume expander P: blood derivative	Albuminar 5%, Albutein 5%, Buminate 5%, Plasbumin 5%
albumin 25% T: plasma volume expander P: blood derivative	Albuminar 25%, Albumisol 25%, Buminate 25%, Plasbumin 25%
albuterol (salbutamol) T: bronchodilator P: adrenergic	Proventil, Respolin‡
albuterol sulfate (salbutamol sulphate) T: bronchodilator P: adrenergic	Proventil, Proventil Repetabs, Respolin Inhaler‡, Respolin Inhaler Solution‡, Ventolin Obstetric Injection‡
alclometasone dipropionate T: anti-inflammatory P: topical adrenocorticoid	Alclovate, Logoderm‡
aldesleukin (interleukin-2) T: immune stimulant P: glycoprotein	Proleukin
alfentanil hydrochloride T: analgesic, adjunct to anesthesia, anesthetic P: opioid	Alfenta
alglucerase (ceramide glucosidase, gluco-cerebrosidase, gluco-sylceramidase, gluco-cerebrosidase-beta-glucosidase) T: replacement enzyme P: glycosidase	Ceredase
allopurinol T: antigout agent P: xanthine oxidase inhibitor	Alloremed‡, Capurate‡, Lopurin, Zyloprim
alpha₁-proteinase inhibitor (human) (alpha₁-PI) T: orphan drug P: enzyme inhibitor	Prolastin
alprazolam T: antianxiety agent P: benzodiazepine	Xanax

T Therapeutic classification.   P Pharmacologic classification.

GENERIC NAME AND CLASSIFICATIONS	TRADE NAMES
alprostadil T: ductus arteriosus patency adjunct P: prostaglandin	Prostin VR Pediatric
alteplase (tissue plasminogen activator, recombinant; t-PA) T: thrombolytic enzyme P: enzyme	Actilyse‡, Activase
altretamine (hexamethylmelamine; HMM) T: antineoplastic P: alkylating agent	Hexalen
aluminum carbonate T: antacid, hypophosphatemic agent P: inorganic aluminum salt	Basaljel
aluminum hydroxide T: antacid, hypophosphatemic agent, adsorbent P: aluminum salt	Algicon*, Alicalade*, Alsorb Gel*, ALternaGEL, Alu-Cap, Aludrox*, Alu-Tab, Amphojel, Amphotabs‡, Antacid G*, Antacid Tabs*, Apcogesic*, Arcodex Antacid*, Ascriptin*, Ascriptin A/D*, Ascriptin Extra Strength*, Ascriptin with Codeine*, Asmadrin*, Azolid-A*, Butazolidin Alicia*, Calciphen*, Cama*, Cama Arthritis Strength*, Camalox*, Delcid*, Di-Gel*, Dialume, Dristan*, Eugel*, Eulcin*, Enterex*, Escot*, Fermalox*, Fernisolone B*, Gacid*, Gas-Eze*, Gaysal-S*, Gaviscon*, Gelusil*, Glycogel*, Kapinal*, Kolantyl*, Maalox*, Maalox Plus*, Magnatril*, Malcogel*, Malcotabs*, Manalum*, Maracaid-2*, Maralen*, Metropectin*, Mucogel*, Mylanta*, Mylanta II*, Nephrox, Neutralox*, Neutrameg*, Predoxide*, Silain Gel*, Silmagel*, Simeco*, Simethox*, Spasmasorb*, Triactin*, Trialka*, Trisogel*, Wingel*
aluminum phosphate T: antacid P: aluminum salt	Phosphaljel

---

† Available in Canada only.   ‡ Available in Australia only.   * Combination product.

GENERIC NAME AND CLASSIFICATIONS	TRADE NAMES
amantadine hydrochloride T: antiviral, antiparkinsonian agent P: synthetic cyclic primary amine	Antadine‡, Symadine, Symmetrel
ambenonium chloride T: antimyasthenic agent P: cholinesterase inhibitor	Mytelase
amcinonide T: anti-inflammatory agent P: topical adrenocorticoid	Cyclocort
amikacin sulfate T: antibiotic P: aminoglycoside	Amikin
amiloride hydrochloride T: diuretic, antihypertensive P: potassium-sparing diuretic	Kaluril‡, Midamor, Moduretic*
amino acid infusions, crystalline T: parenteral nutrition therapy and caloric agent P: protein substrates	Aminosyn, Aminosyn II, Aminosyn-PF, FreAmine III, Geramine*, Novamine, Stuart Amino Acids & B$_{12}$*, Travasol, TrophAmine
amino acid infusions in dextrose T: parenteral nutritional therapy and caloric agent P: protein substrates	Aminosyn II with Dextrose*
amino acid infusions with electrolytes T: parenteral nutritional therapy and caloric agent P: protein substrates	Aminosyn with Electrolytes, Aminosyn II with Electrolytes, FreAmine III with Electrolytes, ProcalAmine with Electrolytes, Travasol with Electrolytes
amino acid infusions with electrolytes in dextrose T: parenteral nutritional therapy and caloric agent P: protein substrates	Aminosyn II with Electrolytes in Dextrose*
amino acid infusions for hepatic failure T: parenteral nutritional therapy and caloric agent P: protein substrates	HepatAmine

T Therapeutic classification.   P Pharmacologic classification.

GENERIC NAME AND CLASSIFICATIONS	TRADE NAMES
amino acid infusions for high metabolic stress T: parenteral nutritional therapy and caloric agent P: protein substrates	Aminosyn-HBC, BranchAmin, FreAmine HBC
amino acid infusions for renal failure T: parenteral nutritional therapy and caloric agent P: protein substrates	Aminess, Aminosyn-RF, NephrAmine, RenAmin
aminocaproic acid T: fibrinolysis inhibitor P: carboxylic acid derivative	Amicar
aminoglutethimide T: antineoplastic P: antiadrenal hormone	Cytadren
aminophylline (theophylline ethylenediamine) T: bronchodilator P: xanthine derivative	Aminophyllin, Amodrine*, Amphedrine Compound*, Asmadrin*, Asminorel*, B.M.E.*, Bronchovent*, Cardophyllin‡, Corophyllin†, Mudrane GG-2*, Neogen*, Phyllocontin, Romaphed*, Somophyllin-DF, Strema*
amiodarone hydrochloride T: ventricular and supraventricular antiarrhythmic P: benzofuran derivative	Cordarone, Cordarone X‡
amitriptyline hydrochloride T: antidepressant P: tricyclic antidepressant	Amitril, Apo-Amitriptyline†, Elavil, Emitrip, Endep, Enovil, Etrafon*, Laroxyl‡, Levate†, Limbitrol*, Meravil†, Novo-Triptyn†, Triavil*
ammonium chloride T: acidifying agent, expectorant P: acid-forming salt	Bentrac Expectorant*, Cheratussin*, Efricon Expectorant*, Eladryl Expectorant*, Fenylex Expectorant*, Formadrin*, Infantuss*, Niltuss*, Partuss*, Quelidrine*, Rinocidin Caps*, Scotuf*, Shertuss*, Thor Syrup*, Tusstat Expectorant*, Zypan*
amobarbital T: sedative-hypnotic, anticonvulsant P: barbiturate	Amodex*, Amoseco*, Amytal Bronchovent*, Dextrobar*, Obe-Slim*, Penta-Cap Plus*, Romaphed*, Scoline Amobarbital*, Trimex*, Tuinal*

---

† Available in Canada only.   ‡ Available in Australia only.   * Combination product.

GENERIC NAME AND CLASSIFICATIONS	TRADE NAMES

amobarbital sodium
T: sedative-hypnotic, anticon-
vulsant
P: barbiturate

Amsee*, Amytal Sodium Broncho-
vent*, Compobarb*, Dusotal*,
Lanabarb*

amoxapine
T: antidepressant
P: dibenzoxazepine, tricyclic
antidepressant

Asendin

**amoxicillin/clavulanate po-
tassium (amoxycillin/
clavulanate potassium)**
T: antibiotic
P: aminopenicillin and beta-
lactamase inhibitor

Augmentin, Clavulin†

**amoxicillin trihydrate
(amoxycillin trihydrate)**
T: antibiotic
P: aminopenicillin

Alphamox‡, Amoxil, Apo-Amoxi†,
Augmentin*, Axicillin†, Cilamox‡,
Ibiamox‡, Moxacin‡, Novamoxin†,
Polymox†, Trimox, Utimox, Wymox

amphetamine sulfate
T: CNS stimulant, short-term
adjunctive anorexigenic
agent, sympathomimetic
amine
P: amphetamine

amphotericin B
T: antifungal
P: polyene macrolide

Fungilin Oral‡, Fungizone, Mysteclin*

ampicillin
T: antibiotic
P: aminopenicillin

Amcill, Ampicin†, Ampilean†, Apo-
Ampi†, Novo Ampicillin†, Omnipen,
Penbritin†, Polycillin PRB*, Principen
Principen with Probenecid*, Pro-
bandacin*

ampicillin sodium
T: antibiotic
P: aminopenicillin

Ampicyn Injection‡, Omnipen-N,
Polycillin-N, Totacillin-N

**ampicillin sodium/sul-
bactam sodium**
T: antibiotic
P: aminopenicillin/beta-
lactamase inhibitor
combination

Unasyn

T Therapeutic classification.   P Pharmacologic classification.

GENERIC NAME AND CLASSIFICATIONS	TRADE NAMES
ampicillin trihydrate T: antibiotic P: aminopenicillin	Amcill, Ampicyn Oral‡, D-Amp, Omnipen, Penamp-250, Penamp-500, Penbritin‡, Polycillin, Principen-250, Principen-500, Probampacin*, Totacillin
amrinone lactate T: inotropic, vasodilator P: bipyridine derivative	Inocor
amsacrine (m-AMSA) T: antineoplastic P: alkylating agent	Amsidyl†
amyl nitrite T: vasodilator, cyanide poisoning adjunct P: nitrate	Cyanide Antidote Package*
anisotropine methylbromide T: antimuscarinic, gastrointestinal antispasmodic P: anticholinergic, synthetic belladonna alkaloid derivative	Valpin 50
anistreplase (anisoylated plasminogen-streptokinase activator complex; APSAC) T: thrombolytic enzyme P: thrombolytic enzyme	Eminase
antihemophilic factor (AHF) T: antihemophilic agent P: blood derivative	Hemofil M, Koate-HS, Monoclate
antirabies serum, equine T: rabies prophylaxis product P: immune serum	
antithrombin III (heparin cofactor I) T: anticoagulant, antithrombotic P: glycoprotein	ATnativ
apomorphine hydrochloride T: emetic P: semisynthetic alkaloidal salt	

---

† Available in Canada only.   ‡ Available in Australia only.   * Combination product.

GENERIC NAME AND CLASSIFICATIONS	TRADE NAMES
apraclonidine hydro-chloride T: ocular hypotensive agent P: alpha-adrenergic agonist	Iopidine
aprobarbital T: sedative-hypnotic P: barbiturate	Alurate
artificial tears T: demulcent P: derivatives of polyvinyl alcohol or cellulose	Adsorbotear, Hypotears, Isopto Alkaline, Isopto Plain, Isopto Tears, Lacril, Lacrisert, Liquifilm Forte, Liquifilm Tears, Lyteers, Methulose, Moisture Drops, Neo-Tears, Refresh, Tearisol, Tears Naturale, Tears Plus, Ultra Tears, Visculose
asparaginase (L-as-paraginase) T: antineoplastic P: enzyme (L-asparagine amidohydrolase, cell cycle–phase specific, G_1 phase)	Elspar, Kidrolase†
aspirin (acetylsalicylic acid) T: nonnarcotic analgesic, antipyretic, anti-inflammatory, antiplatelet P: salicylate	Alka Seltzer*, Alka Seltzer Plus*, Aminodyne*, Ancasal†, A.P.C.*, Arthrinol†, Artria SR, ASA, ASA Comp*, ASA Enseals, Ascriptin*, Ascriptin A/D*, Ascriptin Extra Strength*, Ascriptin with Codeine*, Aspergum, Aspirbar*, Aspirin Plus*, Aspirin with Codeine #2*, Aspirin with Codeine #3*, Aspirin with Codeine #4*, Aspro‡, Astrin†, Axotal*, Bayer Aspirin, Bayer Children's Cold Tabs*, BC Powder*, Bex‡, Buff-A-Comp*, Buff-A-Comp #3*, Buffaprin*, Bufferin*, Bufferin Arthritis Strength*, Bufferin Arthritis Strength Tri-Buff*, Bufferin Extra Strength*, Bufferin Extra Strength Tri-Buff*, Buffinol*, Calciphen*, Cama Arthritis Strength, Coryphen†, Damascon*, Darvon Compound-65*, Darvon with Aspirin*, Dolene Compound-65*, Doloral*, Dolor Plus*, Dorophen Compound-65*, Dristan*, Easprin, Ecotrin, Emagrin*, Empirin, Entrophen†, Excedrin*, Fiorinal*, 4-Way Tabs*, Measurin, Midol*, Nodalin*, Norgesic*, Norgesic Forte*, Norwich Aspirin, Novasen†, PAC*,

GENERIC NAME AND CLASSIFICATIONS	TRADE NAMES
aspirin *(continued)*	Palgesic*, Phenetron Compound*, Presalin*, Riphen-10†, Robaxisal*, Rotenase*, Sal-Adult†, Saleto*, Saleto-D*, Salocol*, Sal-Infant†, Sarogesic*, Sedalgesic*, Sine-Off*, Solprin‡, St. Joseph Cold Tabs*, Supasa†, Triaphen-10†, Trigesic*, Vanquish*, Vincent's Powders‡, Winsprin Capsules‡, Zorprin
astemizole T: antiallergy agent P: histamine₁-receptor antagonist	Hismanal
atenolol T: antihypertensive, antianginal P: beta-adrenergic blocking agent	Noten‡, Tenormin
atracurium besylate T: skeletal muscle relaxant P: nondepolarizing neuromuscular blocking agent	Tracrium
atropine sulfate T: antiarrhythmic, vagolytic P: anticholinergic, belladonna alkaloid	Antrocol*, Atropisol, Atrophysine*, Atropt‡, Azo-Cyst*, Barbeloid*, Brobella-P.B.*, BufOpto Atropine, Butabell HMB*, Capahist-DMH*, Chlorodri*, Coryza*, Cystrea*, Decojen*, Detal*, Dezest*, Diaction*, Donnacin*, Donnatal*, Donnatal #2*, Donnazyme*, Eldonal*, Enterex*, Fenatron*, Fitacol*, Haponal*, Hexalol*, Histapco*, Hyonal C.T.*, Hyonatal*, Hyonatal B-Elixir*, Hytrona*, Isopto Atropine Kaosil*, Kapigam*, Kinesed*, Koryza*, Lanased*, Lomotil*, Magnox*, Mass-Donna*, Motofen*, Nilspasm*, Palbar #2*, Palsorb Improved*, Partuss-A*, Peece Kaps*, Phenahist Injection*, Pyma Injection*, RoTrim*, Scopine*, Sedamine*, Sedapar*, Setamine*, Sidonna*, Spabelin Elixir*, Spasaid*, Spasmolin*, Spasquid*, Stannitol*, Ultabs*, Uriprel*, Urisan-P*, Urised*, Urogesic*

GENERIC NAME AND CLASSIFICATIONS	TRADE NAMES
auranofin T: antiarthritic P: gold salt	Ridaura
aurothioglucose T: antiarthritic P: gold salt	Gold-50‡, Solganal
azacytidine (5-azacytidine) T: antineoplastic P: antimetabolite (cell cycle–phase specific, S phase)	
azatadine maleate T: antihistamine P: piperidine antihistamine	Optimine, Zadine‡
azathioprine T: immunosuppressive P: purine antagonist	Imuran, Thioprine‡
azithromycin T: antibiotic P: azalide macrolide	Zithromax
azlocillin sodium T: antibiotic P: extended-spectrum penicillin, acylaminopenicillin	Azlin, Securopen‡
aztreonam T: antibiotic P: monobactam	Azactam

B

GENERIC NAME AND CLASSIFICATIONS	TRADE NAMES
bacampicillin hydrochloride T: antibiotic P: aminopenicillin	Penglobe†, Spectrobid
bacillus Calmette-Guérin (BCG), live intravesical T: antineoplastic agent P: bacterial agent	TheraCys, TICE BCG
bacillus Calmette-Guérin (BCG) vaccine T: bacterial vaccine P: vaccine	
bacitracin T: antibiotic P: polypeptide antibiotic	Baciguent, Bacimycin Ointment*, Bacitin†, Bacitracin*, Bacitracin Methylene Disalicylate*, Bacitracin Neomycin Ointment*, Baximan Ointment*, Biotic Opthalmic with Hydrocortisone Ointment*, BPN Ointment*, Cortisporin Ophthalmic Ointment*, Epimycin A*, Mycitracin Ointment*, Mity-mycin Ointment*, Neomycin Ointment*, Neomycin Sulfate and Bacitracin Ointment*, Neopolycin-HC Ointment*, Neosporin Ointment*, Neo-Thrycex*, Polysporin*, Polysporin Spray*, Tigo Ointment*, Tri-Biotic Ointment*, Tri-Bow Ointment*, Trimixin*, Triple Ab Ointment*
baclofen T: skeletal muscle relaxant P: chlorophenyl derivative	Lioresal, Lioresal DS
beclomethasone dipropionate T: anti-inflammatory, antiasthmatic P: glucocorticoid	Aldecin Aqueous Nasal Spray‡, Aldecin Inhaler‡, Becloforte Inhaler‡, Beclovent, Beclovent Rotacaps†, Vanceril
beclomethasone dipropionate monohydrate T: anti-inflammatory, antiasthmatic P: glucocorticoid	Aldecin Aqueous Nasal Spray, Beconase AQ Nasal Spray, Beconase Nasal Inhaler, Vancenase AQ Nasal Spray, Vancenase Nasal Inhaler

---

† Available in Canada only.   ‡ Available in Australia only.   * Combination product.

GENERIC NAME AND CLASSIFICATIONS	TRADE NAMES
belladonna leaf T: antimuscarinic, gastrointestinal antispasmodic P: belladonna alkaloid, anticholinergic	Belladonna Tincture USP, Bellafedrol A-H*, Bellergal*, Butibel*, Cafergot P-B*, Decholin-BB*, Gastrolic*, Kapectocin*, Tialka*, Wigrane*, Wyanoids*
benazepril T: antihypertensive P: angiotensin-converting enzyme inhibitor	Lotensin
bendroflumethiazide (bendrofluazide) T: diuretic, antihypertensive P: thiazide diuretic	Aprinox‡, Aprinox-M‡, Benzide†, Naturetin, Naturetin W-K Tab*, Rautrax-N Modified Tab*, Rauzide Tab*
benzalkonium chloride T: surface antiseptic, antimicrobial preservative P: benzoic acid derivative	Acne Drying Lotion*, Allerest Nasal Spray*, Benz-All, Blephamide Ophthalmic Solution*, Dacriose*, Efricel ⅛%*, Econopred, E-Pilo*, Eye Stream, Germicin, Glaucon Solution*, Garamycin Ophthalmic Solution*, Hyamine 3500, Isotraine Ointment*, Medi-Quik*, Mydfrin Ophthalmic*, Otocalm-H Ear Drops*, Otostan HC*, Otrivin, Prefin A Ophthalmic Solution*, Prefin Z Ophthalmic Solution*, Sinarest Aerosol*, Swim-Eye Drops*, Ultra Tears, Unguentine Spray*, Zephiran Chloride Preps
benzocaine T: anesthetic P: local anesthetic (ester)	Aerocaine*, Americaine*, Anocaine*, Biscolan*, Biscolan HC*, Bonate*, Cetacaine*, Derma Medicone-HC*, Dermoplast*, Doctient HC*, Gastrolic*, Neogen*, Pazo*, Rite-Diet*, Spec-T Sore Throat Cough Suppressant Lozenges*, 20-Cain Burn Relief*, Tympagesic*, Vicks Cough Silencers*
benzonatate T: nonnarcotic antitussive agent P: local anesthetic (ester)	Tessalon
benzoyl peroxide cleansers T: antibacterial agent P: benzoic acid derivative	Benzac 5 and 10 Gel*, Benzac W Wash 5, Benzac W Wash 10, Desquam-X 5 Wash, Desquam-X 10 Wash, Desquam-X Gel*, Fostex 10% BPO Cleansing, Fostex 10% BPO Wash, Loroxide-HC Lotion*, Oxy-10 Wash, PanOxyl 5, PanOxyl 10, Propa

GENERIC NAME AND CLASSIFICATIONS	TRADE NAMES
benzoyl peroxide cleansers (*continued*)	P.H. Liquid Acne Soap, Sulfoxyl Lotion*, Vanoxide-HC Lotion*
benzoyl peroxide creams T: antibacterial agent P: benzoic acid derivative	Acne-Aid, Clearasil Maximum Strength, Cuticura Acne, Dry and Clear Double Strength, Fostex 10% BPO Tinted, Oxy 10 Cover, pHisoAc BP, Vanoxide-HC*
benzoyl peroxide gels T: antibacterial agent P: benzoic acid derivative	Ben-Aqua 5, Ben-Aqua 10, 5 Benzagel, 10 Benzagel, Benzac 5, Benzac W 5, Benzac W 10, Benzac W 2½, Buf-Oxal 10, Clear By Design, Del Aqua 5, Del Aqua 10, Desquam-E, Desquam-X 2.5, Desquam-X 5, Desquam-X 10, Fostex 5% BPO, Fostex 10% BPO, PanOxyl 5, PanOxyl 10, PanOxyl AQ 5, PanOxyl AQ 10, PanOxyl AQ 2 1/2, Persa-Gel, Persa-Gel W 5%, Persa-Gel W 10%, Xerac BP5, Xerac BP10, Zeroxin-5, Zeroxin-10
benzoyl peroxide lotions T: antibacterial agent P: benzoic acid derivative	Acne-10, Ben-Aqua 5, Benoxyl 5, Benoxyl 10, Clearasil 10, Dry and Clear, Loroxide , Oxy 5, Oxy 10, Vanoxide
benzphetamine hydrochloride T: short-term adjunctive anorexigenic agent for refractory exogenous obesity, sympathomimetic amine P: amphetamine	Didrex
benzquinamide hydrochloride T: antiemetic P: benzoquinolizine derivative	Emete-Con
benzthiazide T: diuretic, antihypertensive P: thiazide diuretic	Aquatag, Exna, Hydrex, Proaqua
benztropine mesylate T: antiparkinsonian agent P: anticholinergic	Apo-Benztropine†, Bensylate†, Cogentin, Cogentin Tap Amp*, PMS Benztropine†
benzyl benzoate lotion T: antibacterial agent P: benzoic acid derivative	Scabanca†

---

† Available in Canada only.   ‡ Available in Australia only.   * Combination product.

GENERIC NAME AND CLASSIFICATIONS	TRADE NAMES
bepridil hydrochloride T: antianginal P: calcium channel blocker	Vascor
beractant (natural lung surfactant) T: lung surfactant P: bovine lung extract	Survanta
betamethasone T: anti-inflammatory P: glucocorticoid	Betnelan†, Celestone
betamethasone acetate and betamethasone sodium phosphate T: anti-inflammatory P: glucocorticoid	Celestone Chronodose‡, Celestone Soluspan
betamethasone benzoate T: anti-inflammatory P: topical glucocorticoid	Benisone, Uticort
betamethasone dipropionate T: anti-inflammatory P: topical glucocorticoid	Alphatrex, Diprolene, Diprolene AF, Diprosone
betamethasone sodium phosphate T: anti-inflammatory P: glucocorticoid	Betameth, Betnesol†, B.S.P., Celestone Phosphate, Cel-U-Jec, Prelestone, Selestoject
betamethasone valerate T: anti-inflammatory P: topical glucocorticoid	Betatrex, Beta-Val, Betnovate‡, Valisone
betaxolol hydrochloride T: antiglaucoma agent, antihypertensive P: beta-adrenergic blocking agent	Betoptic, Kerlone
bethanechol chloride T: urinary tract and gastrointestinal tract stimulant P: cholinergic agonist	Duvoid, Urabeth, Urecholine, Urocarb Liquid‡, Urocarb Tablets‡
biperiden hydrochloride T: antiparkinsonian agent P: anticholinergic	Akineton

GENERIC NAME AND CLASSIFICATIONS	TRADE NAMES
biperiden lactate T: antiparkinsonian agent P: anticholinergic	Akineton Lactate
bisacodyl T: stimulant laxative P: diphenylmethane derivative	Bisacolax†, Bisalax‡, Bisco-Lax, Dacodyl, Deficol, Dulcolax, Durolax‡, Fleet Bisacodyl, Laxit†, Theralax
bismuth subgallate T: antidiarrheal P: adsorbent	Anocaine*, Anugestic*, Anulan*, Anusol*, Anusol HC*, Biscolan*, Bonate*, Cholatabs*, Devrom, Diastay*, Doctient HC*, Kaocasil*, Pile-Gon*, Versal*, Xylocaine Suppositories*
bismuth subsalicylate T: antidiarrheal P: adsorbent	Maximum Strength Pepto-Bismol Liquid, Pepto-Bismol*, Wescola*
bitolterol mesylate T: bronchodilator P: adrenergic, beta$_2$ agonist	Tornalate
black widow spider (*Latrodectus mactans*) antivenin T: black widow spider antivenin P: antivenin	
bleomycin sulfate T: antineoplastic P: antibiotic, antineoplastic (cell cycle–phase specific, G$_2$ and M phase)	Blenoxane
boric acid T: topical anti-infective P: acid	Anocaine*, Anulan*, Aurocaine 2, Auro-Dri, Blinx, Bonate*, Collyrium, Dacriose*, Dri/Ear, Ear-Dry, Mass pH Powder*, M-Z Drops*, Neo-Flo, Phenylzin*, Saratoga Ointment*, Swim Ear Drops*, Versal*, Wyanoids*, Wyanoids HC*
botulinum toxin type A T: muscle relaxant P: neurotoxin	Oculinum
botulism antitoxin, trivalent (ABE) equine T: botulism antitoxin P: antitoxin	

---

† Available in Canada only.   ‡ Available in Australia only.   * Combination product.

GENERIC NAME AND CLASSIFICATIONS	TRADE NAMES
bretylium tosylate T: ventricular antiarrhythmic P: adrenergic blocking agent	Bretylate†‡, Bretylol
bromocriptine mesylate T: semisynthetic ergot alkaloid, dopaminergic agonist, antiparkinsonian agent, inhibitor of prolactin release, inhibitor of growth hormone release P: dopamine receptor agonist	Parlodel
brompheniramine maleate T: antihistamine (H_1-receptor antagonist) P: alkylamine antihistamine	Bro-Expectorant with Codeine*, Brombay, Bromepaph*, Bromphen, Bro-Tane Expectorant*, Chlorphed, Codimal-A, Conjec-B, Cophene-B, Cortane*, Dehist, Diamine TD, Dimetane, Dimetane Decongestant*, Dimetane Expectorant*, Dimetane Expectorant- DC*, Dimetane Extentabs*, Dimetane-Ten, Eldatap*, Histaject Modified, Nasahist B, ND-Stat Revised, Oraminic II, Sinusol-B, Veltane
buclizine hydrochloride T: antiemetic and antivertigo agent P: piperazine-derivative antihistamine	Bucladin-S
bumetanide T: diuretic P: loop diuretic	Bumex, Burinex‡
bupivacaine hydrochloride T: local anesthetic, amide type P: sodium channel blocker	Marcain‡, Marcaine, Sensorcaine
buprenorphine hydrochloride T: analgesic P: narcotic agonist-antagonist, opioid partial agonist	Buprenex, Temgesic Injection‡
bupropion hydrochloride T: antidepressant P: aminoketone	Wellbutrin

GENERIC NAME AND CLASSIFICATIONS	TRADE NAMES
buspirone hydrochloride T: antianxiety agent P: azaspirodecanedione derivative	BuSpar
busulfan T: antineoplastic P: alkylating agent (cell cycle–phase nonspecific)	Myleran
butabarbital sodium T: sedative-hypnotic P: barbiturate	Amino-Bar*, Axotal*, Bancaps*, Banesin Forte*, Barbased, Bisalate*, Bontril*, Buff-A-Comp*, Butabell-HMB*, Butalan, Butibel*, Buticaps, Butisol, Cystospaz-SR*, Day-Barb†, Decholin-BB*, Dilorbron*, Dolor Plus*, Dularin-TH*, Eulcin*, Fiorinal*, Hyonatol*, Hyonatol B Elixir*, Indogesic*, Medihaler-Iso*, Metrogesic*, Minotal*, Monosyl*, Nidar*, Nitrodyl-B*, Nitrotym-Plus*, Pedo-Sol Elixir*, Phrenilin*, Pyridium-Plus*, Quad-Set*, Quiebel*, Sarisol No. 2, Sedragesic*, Sidonna*, Span-RD*, Trio-Bar*
butalbital T: sedative P: barbiturate	Amaphen*, Bancaps*, Buff-A-Comp #3, Dengesic*, Esgic*, Fiorinal*, Fiorinal with Codeine*, Lotusate, Phrenicin*, Phrenicin Forte*, Repan*, Sandoptal, Scotgesic*, Triapin*, Two-Dyne*
butoconazole nitrate T: topical fungistat P: synthetic imidazole derivative	Femstat
butorphanol tartrate T: analgesic, adjunct to anesthesia P: narcotic agonist-antagonist; opioid partial agonist	Stadol

C

GENERIC NAME AND CLASSIFICATIONS	TRADE NAMES
caffeine T: central nervous system stimulant, analeptic, respiratory stimulant P: methylxanthine	Akes-n-Pain*, Amaphen*, Aminodyne*, Anodynos Forte*, A.P.C.*, Aspirin Plus*, Buff-A-Comp*, Buff-A-Comp #3*, Buffaprin*, Buffinol*, Cafergot*, Cafergot-PB*, Caffedrine , Centuss*, Damascon-P*, Darvon Compound-65*, Dexitac, Dolene Compound-65*, Dolor Plus*, Doraphen Compound-65*, Drinophen*, Dristan*, Dularin-TH*, Emagrin*, Emagrin Forte*, Emagrin Professional Strength*, Ergotatropin*, Excedrin*, Fendol*, Fiorinal*, Fiorinal with Codeine*, Histapco*, Histosal #2*, Hycomine Compound*, Midol*, Migral*, Nodalin*, No Doz, Norgesic*, Norgesic Forte*, PAC*, Palgesic*, Partuss-A*, Phenetron Compound*, Phrenicin*, Pyranistan Compound*, Quick Pep , Renpap*, Repan*, Rotenase*, S.A.C. Sinus*, Saleto*, Saleto-D*, Salocol*, Sedacaine*, Statomin Maleate II*, Tirend, Trigesic*, Two-Dyne*, Valihist*, Vanquish*, Vivarin, Wigrane*
calcifediol T: antihypocalcemic P: vitamin D analog	Calderol
calcitonin (human) T: hypocalcemic P: thyroid hormone	Cibacalcin
calcitonin (salmon) T: hypocalcemic P: thyroid hormone	Calcimar, Miacalcin
calcitriol (1,25-dihydroxy-cholecalciferol) T: antihypocalcemic P: vitamin D analog	Rocaltrol

GENERIC NAME AND CLASSIFICATIONS	TRADE NAMES
calcium acetate T: antihyperphosphatemic P: calcium salt	Phos-Ex, Phos-Lo
calcium carbonate T: antacid P: calcium salt	Alkalade*, Alka-Mints, Alkets*, Amitone, Anti-Acid #1*, Apcogesic*, Bufferin Arthritis Strength Tri-Buff*, Bufferin Extra Strength Tri-Buff*, Cal Carb-HD, Calcilac, Calcimax‡, Calglycine, Cal-Plus*, Cal-Sup‡, Camalox*, Chooz, Co-Gel*, Diatrol*, Dicarbosil, Dimacid*, Effercal-600‡, Eligel*, Equilet, Gas-Eze*, Genalac, Glycate, Glycogel*, Gustalac, Kanalka*, Kaocasil*, Kaosil*, Lacto-cal*, Mallamint, Natabec*, Pama No. 1, Pentids*, Pentids 400*, Pentids 800*, Pepto-Bismol*, Rolaids Calcium Rich, Titracid, Titralic*, Tums, Tums E-X Extra Strength, Tums Extra Strength, Tums Liquid Extra Strength
calcium chloride T: therapeutic agent for electrolyte balance, cardiotonic P: calcium supplement	
calcium citrate T: therapeutic agent for electrolyte balance, cardiotonic P: calcium supplement	Citracal
calcium glubionate T: therapeutic agent for electrolyte balance, cardiotonic P: calcium supplement	Neo-Calglucon
calcium gluceptate T: therapeutic agent for electrolyte balance, cardiotonic P: calcium supplement	
calcium gluconate T: therapeutic agent for electrolyte balance, cardiotonic P: calcium supplement	Akes-n-Pain*, Kalcinate, Sedacane*
calcium lactate T: therapeutic agent for electrolyte balance, cardiotonic P: calcium supplement	Calpholac*, Calphosan*, Gylanphen*, Nycralan*, Pergrava #2*, Theola-phen*, Zinc-220*

† Available in Canada only.   ‡ Available in Australia only.   * Combination product.

GENERIC NAME AND CLASSIFICATIONS	TRADE NAMES
calcium phosphate, dibasic T: therapeutic agent for electrolyte balance, cardiotonic P: calcium supplement	
calcium phosphate, tribasic T: therapeutic agent for electrolyte balance, cardiotonic P: calcium supplement	Posture
calcium polycarbophil T: bulk laxative, antidiarrheal P: hydrophilic agent	Equalactin, FiberCon, Mitrolan
capreomycin sulfate T: antitubercular agent P: polypeptide antibiotic	Capastat
capsaicin T: topical analgesic P: substance-P antagonist	Axsain, Zostrix
captopril T: antihypertensive, adjunctive treatment of congestive heart failure P: angiotensin-converting enzyme inhibitor	Capoten
carbachol (intraocular) T: miotic P: cholinergic agonist	Isopto Carbachol*, Miostat
carbachol (topical) T: miotic P: cholinergic agonist	Carbacel, Isopto Carbachol Solution*
carbamazepine T: anticonvulsant, analgesic P: iminostilbene derivative; chemically related to tricyclic antidepressants	Apo-Carbamazepine†, Epitol, Mazepine†, Tegretol, Tegretol CR†, Teril‡
carbamide peroxide T: ceruminolytic, topical antiseptic P: urea hydrogen peroxide	Debrox
carbenicillin disodium T: antibiotic P: extended-spectrum penicillin, alpha-carboxypenicillin	Carbapen‡, Geopen, Pyopen

T Therapeutic classification.   P Pharmacologic classification.

GENERIC NAME AND CLASSIFICATIONS	TRADE NAMES
carbenicillin indanyl sodium T: antibiotic P: extended-spectrum penicillin, alpha-carboxypenicillin	Geocillin, Geopen Oral†
carbidopa-levodopa T: antiparkinsonian agent P: decarboxylase inhibitor–dopamine precursor combination	Sinemet
carbol-fuchsin solution (Castellani's paint; Magenta paint) T: topical antifungal P: aniline derivative	Castaderm
carboplatin T: antineoplastic P: alkylating agent (cell cycle–phase nonspecific)	Paraplatin
carboprost tromethamine T: oxytocic P: prostaglandin	Hemabate, Prostin/15 M
carisoprodol T: skeletal muscle relaxant P: carbamate derivative	Rela, Sodol, Soma, Soprodol, Soridol
carmustine (BCNU) T: antineoplastic P: alkylating agent; nitrosourea (cell cycle–phase nonspecific)	BiCNU
carteolol hydrochloride T: antihypertensive P: beta-adrenergic blocking agent	Cartrol
casanthranol T: cathartic P: anthranol glycoside	Black Draught, Calotabs*, Constiban*, Dialose Plus*, Diolax*, Dio-Soft*, Disanthrol*, Disolam Forte*, Di-Sosul Forte*, Easy Lax Plus*, Genericace*, Neo-Vadrin D-D-S*, Nuvac*, Peri-Colace*, Rodox*, Tri-Vac*

† Available in Canada only.   ‡ Available in Australia only.   * Combination product.

GENERIC NAME AND CLASSIFICATIONS	TRADE NAMES
cascara sagrada T: laxative P: anthraquinone glycoside mixture	Cas-Evac, Nature's Remedy
castor oil T: stimulant laxative P: glyceride, *Ricinus communis* derivative	Alphamul, Emulsoil, Fleet Flavored Castor Oil, Kellogg's Castor Oil, Minims Castor Oil‡, Neoloid, Purge
cefaclor T: antibiotic P: second-generation cephalosporin	Ceclor
cefadroxil monohydrate T: antibiotic P: first-generation cephalosporin	Duricef, Ultracef
cefamandole nafate T: antibiotic P: second-generation cephalosporin	Mandol
cefazolin sodium T: antibiotic P: first-generation cephalosporin	Ancef, Kefzol
cefixime T: antibiotic P: third-generation cephalosporin	Suprax
cefmetazole sodium T: antibiotic P: second-generation cephalosporin	Zefazone
cefonicid sodium T: antibiotic P: second-generation cephalosporin	Monocid
cefoperazone sodium T: antibiotic P: third-generation cephalosporin	Cefobid
ceforanide T: antibiotic P: second-generation cephalosporin	Precef

T Therapeutic classification.   P Pharmacologic classification.

GENERIC NAME AND CLASSIFICATIONS	TRADE NAMES
cefotaxime sodium T: antibiotic P: third-generation cephalosporin	Claforan
cefotetan disodium T: antibiotic P: second-generation cephalosporin, cephamycin	Cefotan
cefoxitin sodium T: antibiotic P: second-generation cephalosporin, cephamycin	Mefoxin
cefprozil monohydrate T: antibiotic P: second-generation cephalosporin	Cefzil
ceftazidime T: antibiotic P: third-generation cephalosporin	Fortaz, Magnacef†, Tazicef, Tazidime
ceftizoxime sodium T: antibiotic P: third-generation cephalosporin	Cefizox
ceftriaxone sodium T: antibiotic P: third-generation cephalosporin	Rocephin
cefuroxime axetil T: antibiotic P: second-generation cephalosporin	Ceftin
cefuroxime sodium T: antibiotic P: second-generation cephalosporin	Kefurox, Zinacef
cephalexin monohydrate T: antibiotic P: first-generation cephalosporin	Ceporex†‡, Keflet, Keflex, Keftab, Novolexin†
cephalothin sodium T: antibiotic P: first-generation cephalosporin	Ceporacin†‡, Keflin

† Available in Canada only.   ‡ Available in Australia only.   * Combination product.

GENERIC NAME AND CLASSIFICATIONS	TRADE NAMES
cephapirin sodium T: antibiotic P: first-generation cephalosporin	Cefadyl
cephradine T: antibiotic P: first-generation cephalosporin	Anspor, Velosef
chenodiol (chenodeoxycholic acid) T: cholelitholytic P: bile acid	Chenix
chloral hydrate T: sedative-hypnotic P: general central nervous system depressant	Aquachloral Supprettes, Noctec, Novochlorhydrate†
chlorambucil T: antineoplastic P: alkylating agent (cell cycle–phase nonspecific)	Leukeran
chloramphenicol T: antibiotic P: dichloroacetic acid derivative	AK-Chlor, Chloromycetin Ophthalmic, Chloromyxin Opthalmic Ointment*, Chloromycetin, Chloroptic, Chloroptic S.O.P., Chlorsig‡, Fenicol†, Isopto Fenicol†, Novochlorocap†, Ophthoclor Ophthalmic, Opthocort*, Pentamycetin†, Sopamycetin†
chloramphenicol palmitate T: antibiotic P: dichloroacetic acid derivative	Chloromycetin Palmitate
chloramphenicol sodium succinate T: antibiotic P: dichloroacetic acid derivative	Chloromycetin Sodium Succinate, Pentamycetin†
chlordiazepoxide T: antianxiety agent; anticonvulsant; sedative-hypnotic P: benzodiazepine	Libritabs, Limbitrol*

T Therapeutic classification.   P Pharmacologic classification.

GENERIC NAME AND CLASSIFICATIONS	TRADE NAMES
chlordiazepoxide hydrochloride T: antianxiety agent; anticonvulsant; sedative-hypnotic P: benzodiazepine	Apo-Chlordiazepoxide†, Librax*, Librium, Lipoxide, Medilium†, Mitran, Novopoxide†, Reposans, Sereen, Solium
chloroprocaine hydrochloride T: local anesthetic, amide derivative P: sodium channel blocker	Nesacaine, Nesacaine MPF
chloroquine hydrochloride T: antimalarial, amebicide, anti-inflammatory P: 4-aminoquinoline	Aralen HCl, Chlorquin‡
chloroquine phosphate T: antimalarial, amebicide, anti-inflammatory P: 4-aminoquinoline	Aralen Phosphate, Chlorquin‡
chloroquine sulphate T: antimalarial P: aminoquinolone derivative	Nivaquine‡
chlorothiazide T: diuretic, antihypertensive P: thiazide diuretic	Aldoclor*, Azide‡, Chlotride‡, Diachlor, Diupres*, Diuret‡, Diurigen, Diuril
chlorothiazide sodium T: diuretic, antihypertensive P: thiazide diuretic	Diuril Sodium
chlorotrianisene T: estrogen relacement, antineoplastic P: estrogen	Tace
chlorphenesin carbamate T: skeletal muscle relaxant P: carbamate derivative	Maolate
chlorpheniramine maleate T: antihistamine (H_1-receptor antagonist) P: propylamine-derivative antihistamine	Al-Ay*, Alka-Seltzer*, Aller-Chlor, Allerdec*, Allergex‡, Alumadrine*, Anodynos Forte*, A.R.M.*, Atussin*, Atussin DM*, BC-Powder*, Bellafedrol A-H*, B.M.E. Liquid*, Bobid*, B.Q. Cold*, Breacol*, Brolade*, Bur-Tuss*, Capahist-DMH*, CDM Expectorant*, Centuss*, Cerose-DM*, Chew-Hist*, Chlo-Amine, Chlo- *(continued)*

GENERIC NAME AND CLASSIFICATIONS	TRADE NAMES

chlorpheniramine maleate
(continued)

rate, Chlor-Niramine, Chlorodri*, Chlor-100, Chlor-Pro, Chlor-Pro 10, Chlorspan-12, Chlortab-4, Chlortab-8, Chlor-Trimeton, Chlor-Trimeton Repetabs, Chlor-Tripolon, Codimal*, Colrex Compound*, Colrex Syrup*, Comtrex*, Conalsyn*, Contac 12 Hour*, Cophene #2*, Cophene-PL*, Cophene-S*, Cophene-X*, Corcidin Sinus Headache*, Corilin*, Co-Tylenol*, Dallergy*, Decobel*, Decojen*, Deconamine*, Dehist*, Demazin*, Derma-Pax*, Dezest*, Donatussin*, Dristan 12 Hour*, Drucon*, Efricon Expectorant*, Extendryl*, Fedahist*, F.C.A.H.*, Fitacol*, Formadrin*, 4-Way Tab*, Genallerate, Guistrey Fortis*, Histacon*, Histapco*, Histaspan-D*, Histaspan Plus*, Hista-Vadrin*, Histogesic*, Histone*, Hycoff-A*, Hycomine Compound*, Infantuss*, Kiddies Sialco*, Koryza*, Kronofed-A*, Lanatuss*, Marhist*, Nasahist Caps*, N-D Gesic*, Nilcol*, Niltuss*, Nolamine*, Novafed A*, Novahistine DH*, Novopheniram‡, Partuss*, Pediacof*, Pedosol Elixir*, Pfeiffer's Allergy, Phenahist Injection*, Phenahist-TR Tabs*, Phenatuss Expectorant*, Phenetron, Phenetron Compound*, Piriton‡, P.M.P. Expectorant*, Polytuss-DM*, Pyma*, Pyma Injection*, Pyranistan, Pyranistan Compound*, Pyranistan Syrup*, Pyristan*, Quelidrine Syrup*, Rentuss*, Rhiney*, Rhinogesic*, Rinocidin Caps*, Rinocidin Expectorant*, Rohist-D Expectorant*, Rolanade*, Ryna*, Ryna-C*, Salphenyl*, Santussin*, Scotuss*, Scotcof*, Scotnord*, Shertuss Liquid*, Sialco*, Sinarest*, Sine-Off*, Sinovan Timed*, Sinucol*, Sinulin*, Sinutab*, Spantuss*, Statomin Maleate II*, Sudafed Plus*, Symptrol*, Telachlor, Teldrin, Theospaw*, Tonecol Cough Syrup*, Triaminic Cold Syrup*, Triaminic Cold Tabs*, Triaminicin*, Triaminic Multi-Symptom Cold Syrup*, Triami-

---

T Therapeutic classification.   P Pharmacologic classification.

GENERIC NAME AND CLASSIFICATIONS	TRADE NAMES
chlorpheniramine maleate *(continued)*	nic Multi-Symptom Cold Tablets*, Triaminic Nite Light Cold*, Triaminic-12 Tabs*, Trigelamine*, Tri-Histin Expectorant*, Trind- DM*, Trymegen, Turbilixir*, Turbispan Leisurecaps*, Tusquelin*, Tussafed Expectorant*, Tussar-2 Syrup*, Tussar-DM*, Tussar-SF*, Valihist*, Wal-Phed Plus*
chlorpromazine hydrochloride T: antipsychotic, antiemetic P: aliphatic phenothiazine	Chlorpromanyl†, Largactil†‡, Novo-Chlorpromazine†, Protran‡, Thorazine, Thor-Pram
chlorpropamide T: antidiabetic agent, antidiuretic agent P: sulfonylurea	Apo-Chlorpropamide†, Diabinese, Glucamide, Novo-propamide†
chlorprothixene T: antipsychotic P: thioxanthene	Taractan, Tarasan†
chlortetracycline hydrochloride T: antibiotic, anti-infective P: tetracycline	Aureomycin 3%
chlorthalidone T: diuretic, antihypertensive P: thiazide-like diuretic	Apo-Chlorthalidone†, Demi-Regroton*, Hygroton, Novothalidone†, Regroton*, Thalitone, Uridon†
chlorzoxazone T: skeletal muscle relaxant P: benzoxazole derivative	Blanex*, Paraflex, Parafon Forte DSC*, Strifon Forte DSC
cholera vaccine T: cholera prophylaxis product P: vaccine	
cholestyramine T: antilipemic, bile acid sequestrant P: anion exchange resin	Cholybar, Questran
choline magnesium trisalicylate (choline salicylate and magnesium salicylate) T: nonnarcotic analgesic, antipyretic, anti-inflammatory P: salicylate	Trilisate

† Available in Canada only.   ‡ Available in Australia only.   * Combination product.

GENERIC NAME AND CLASSIFICATIONS	TRADE NAMES
choline salicylate T: nonnarcotic analgesic, antipyretic, anti-inflammatory P: salicylate	Arthropan, Teejel†
chymopapain T: chemonucleolytic agent P: proteolytic enzyme	Chymodiactin, Discase
ciclopirox olamine T: topical antifungal P: N-hydroxypyridinone derivative	Loprox
cimetidine T: antiulcer agent P: histamine$_2$-receptor antagonist	Doractin‡, Tagamet
cinoxacin T: urinary tract antiseptic P: quinolone antibiotic	Cinobac
ciprofloxacin T: antibiotic P: quinolone antibiotic	Cipro, Cipro I.V., Ciproxin‡
cisplatin (cis-platinum) T: antineoplastic P: alkylating agent (cell cycle–phase nonspecific)	Platamine‡, Platinol
clarithromycin T: antibiotic P: macrolide	Zithromax
clemastine fumarate T: antihistamine (H$_1$-receptor antagonist) P: ethanolamine-derivative antihistamine	Tavist, Tavist-1
clidinium bromide T: antimuscarinic, gastrointestinal antispasmodic P: anticholinergic	Librax*, Quarzan
clindamycin hydrochloride T: antibiotic P: lincomycin derivative	Cleocin HCl, Dalacin C‡

T Therapeutic classification.   P Pharmacologic classification.

GENERIC NAME AND CLASSIFICATIONS	TRADE NAMES
clindamycin palmitate hydrochloride T: antibiotic P: lincomycin derivative	Cleocin Pediatric, Dalacin C Palmitate‡
clindamycin phosphate T: antibiotic P: lincomycin derivative	Cleocin, Cleocin Phosphate, Cleocin T Gel (Lotion, Solution), Dalacin C†‡, Dalacin C Phosphate
clobetasol propionate T: anti-inflammatory P: topical adrenocorticoid	Dermovate†, Temovate
clocortolone pivalate T: anti-inflammatory P: topical adrenocorticoid	Cloderm
clofazimine T: leprostatic P: substituted iminophenazine dye	Lamprene
clofibrate T: antilipemic P: fibric acid derivative	Arterioflexin‡, Atromid-S, Claripex†, Novofibrate†
clomiphene citrate T: ovulation stimulant P: chlorotrianisene derivate	Clomid
clomipramine hydrochloride T: antiobsessional agent P: tricyclic antidepressant	Anafranil
clonazepam T: anticonvulsant P: benzodiazepine	Klonopin, Rivotril
clonidine hydrochloride T: antihypertensive P: centrally acting antiadrenergic agent	Catapres, Catapres-TTS, Dixarit†‡
clorazepate dipotassium T: antianxiety agent; anticonvulsant; sedative-hypnotic P: benzodiazepine	Gen-Xene, Novoclopate†, Tranxene, Tranxene-SD, Tranxene-T-Tab
clotrimazole T: topical antifungal P: synthetic imidazole derivative	Canesten†, Gyne-Lotrimin, Lotrimin, Mycelex, Mycelex-G

---

† Available in Canada only.   ‡ Available in Australia only.   * Combination product.

GENERIC NAME AND CLASSIFICATIONS	TRADE NAMES

cloxacillin sodium
T: antibiotic
P: penicillinase-resistant penicillin

Alclox‡, Apo-Cloxi†, Austrastaph‡, Bactopen†, Cloxapen, Novocloxin†, Orbenin†, Orbenin Injection‡, Tegopen

clozapine
T: antipsychotic
P: tricyclic dibenzodiazepine derivative

Clozaril

coccidioidin
T: skin test antigen
P: *Coccidioides immitis* antigen

Spherulin

codeine phosphate
T: analgesic, antitussive
P: opioid

Acetaminophen with Codeine*, Actifed-C Syrup*, Ascriptin with Codeine*, Aspirin with Codeine #2*, Aspirin with Codeine #3*, Aspirin with Codeine #4*, Bancaps*, Codalan*, Colrex Compound*, Co-Xan*, Dimetane Expectorant-DC*, Efricon Expectorant*, Guiatuss DAC Syrup*, Guiatussin with Codeine*, Isoclor Expectorant*, Novahistine DH*, Novahistine Expectorant*, Paveral†, Pediacof*, Phenaphen #2*, Phenaphen #3*, Phenaphen #4*, Phenaphen-650*, Phenatuss*, Phenegran-VC Expectorant*, Phrenicin with Codeine*, P.M.P. Expectorant*, Polyectin*, Proclan Expectorant with Codeine*, Proclan VC Expectorant with Codeine*, Proval #3*, Rinocidin Expectorant*, Robitussin AC*, Robitussin DAC*, Rolamethazine VC Expectorant with Codeine*, Rolamethazine with Codeine*, Ryna-C*, Tolu-Sed*, Triaminic Expectorant with Codeine*, TSG Croup Liquid*, Tussar SF*, Tussar-2 Syrup*, Tylenol with Codeine*

codeine sulfate
T: analgesic, antitussive
P: opioid

Copavin*, Copavin Compound*, Golacol*

colchicine
T: antigout
P: *Colchicum autumnale* alkaloid

Apcogesic*, Benn-C Tab*, Bricolide*, Colbenemid*, Colchicine MR‡, Colgout‡, Colsalide*, Doloral*, Novocolchicine†, Robenecid with Colchicine*, Salcoce*

T Therapeutic classification.   P Pharmacologic classification.

GENERIC NAME AND CLASSIFICATIONS	TRADE NAMES
colestipol hydrochloride T: antilipemic P: anion exchange resin	Colestid
colfosceril palmitate T: lung surfactant P: phospholipid	Exosurf Neonatal
colistimethate sodium (poly-myxin E) T: antibiotic P: polymyxin antibiotic	Coly-Mycin M Parenteral
colistin sulfate T: antibiotic P: polymyxin antibiotic	Coly-Mycin S
corn oil T: enteral nutritional therapy P: modular supplement	Lipomul
corticotropin (adreno-corticotropic hormone, ACTH) T: diagnostic aid, replacement hormone, treatment for multiple sclerosis and non-suppurative thyroiditis P: anterior pituitary hormone	ACTH, Acthar, Acthar Gel (H.P.)†, ACTH Gel, Cortigel-40, Cortigel-80, Cortrophin Gel, Cortropic-Gel-40, Cortropic-Gel-80, H.P. Acthar Gel
cortisone acetate T: anti-inflammatory, replacement therapy P: glucocorticoid, mineralocorticoid	Cortate‡, Cortone Acetate
cosyntropin T: diagnostic agent P: anterior pituitary hormone	Cortrosyn
co-trimoxazole (sul-famethoxazole-trimethoprim) T: antibiotic P: sulfonamide and folate antagonist	Apo-Sulfatrim†, Apo-Sulfatrim DS†, Bactrim, Bactrim DS, Bactrim I.V. Infusion, Cotrim, Cotrim D.S., Novotrimel, Novotrimel DS†, Protrin†, Protrin DF†, Resprim‡, Roubac†, Roubac DS†, Septra, Septra DS, Septra I.V. Infusion, Septrin‡, SMZ-TMP, Sulfamethoprim, Sulfamethoprim DS, Sulmeprim, Trib‡, Uroplus DS, Uroplus SS
cromolyn sodium T: mast cell stabilizer P: chromone derivative	Opticrom 4%

---

† Available in Canada only.   ‡ Available in Australia only.   * Combination product.

GENERIC NAME AND CLASSIFICATIONS	TRADE NAMES
cromolyn sodium (sodium cromoglycate) T: mast cell stabilizer, anti-asthmatic P: chromone derivative	Gastrocrom, Intal, Intal Inhaler, Intal Spincaps†, Nalcrom, Nasalcrom, Op-ticrom, Rynacrom†
crotaline (*Crotalidae*) anti-venin, polyvalent T: snake antivenin P: antivenin	
crotamiton T: scabicide and antipruritic P: synthetic chloroformate salt	Eurax
cyclandelate T: antispasmodic, vasodilator P: mandelic acid derivative	Cyclan, Cyclospasmol
cyclizine hydrochloride T: antiemetic and antivertigo agent P: piperazine-derivative anti-histamine	Marezine, Migral*
cyclizine lactate T: antiemetic and antivertigo agent P: piperazine-derivative anti-histamine	Marezine, Marzine†
cyclobenzaprine T: skeletal muscle relaxant P: tricyclic antidepressant derivative	Flexeril
cyclopentolate hydrochlo-ride T: cycloplegic, mydriatic P: anticholinergic agent	AK-Pentolate, Cyclogyl, Cyclomydril Solution*
cyclophosphamide T: antineoplastic P: alkylating agent (cell cycle–phase nonspecific)	Cycoblastin‡, Cytoxan, Cytoxan Ly-ophilized, Endoxan-Asta‡, Neosar, Procytox†
cycloserine T: antitubercular agent P: isoxizolidone, d-alanine analog	Seromycin

GENERIC NAME AND CLASSIFICATIONS	TRADE NAMES
cyclosporine (cyclosporin) T: immunosuppressant P: polypeptide antibiotic	Sandimmun‡, Sandimmune
cyproheptadine hydrochloride T: antihistamine (H_1-receptor antagonist), antipruritic agent P: piperidine-antihistamine derivative	Periactin
cytarabine (ARA-C, cytosine arabinoside) T: antineoplastic P: antimetabolite (cell cycle–phase specific, S phase)	Alexan‡, Cytosar-U
cytomegalovirus immune globulin (CMV-IGIV, cytomegalovirus immune serum intravenous [human], CytoMune-IV) T: immune serum P: immune globulin	CytoGam

D

GENERIC NAME AND CLASSIFICATIONS	TRADE NAMES
dacarbazine (DTIC) T: antineoplastic P: alkylating agent (cell–cycle phase nonspecific)	DTIC-Dome
dactinomycin (actinomycin D) T: antineoplastic P: antibiotic antineoplastic (cell cycle–phase nonspecific)	Cosmegen
danazol T: antiestrogen, androgen P: androgen	Cyclomen†, Danocrine
dantrolene sodium T: skeletal muscle relaxant P: hydantoin derivative	Dantrium, Dantrium I.V.
dapiprazole hydrochloride T: mydriatic reversal agent P: alpha-adrenergic blocking agent	Rēv-Eyes
dapsone T: antileprotic, antimalarial agent P: synthetic sulfone	Avlosulfon†, Dapsone 100‡
daunorubicin hydrochloride (DNR) T: antineoplastic P: antibiotic antineoplastic (cell cycle–phase nonspecific)	Cerubidin‡, Cerubidine
deferoxamine mesylate T: heavy metal antagonist P: chelating agent	Desferal
dehydrocholic acid T: laxative P: bile acid	Antrocholin, Cholan-DH, Decholin, Hepahydrin
demecarium bromide T: miotic P: cholinesterase inhibitor	Humorsol

T Therapeutic classification.   P Pharmacologic classification.

GENERIC NAME AND CLASSIFICATIONS	TRADE NAMES
demeclocycline hydrocholoride T: antibiotic P: tetracycline antibiotic	Declomycin, Ledermycin‡
deserpidine T: antihypertensive, antipsychotic P: rauwolfia alkaloid, peripherally acting adrenergic-blocking agent	Enduronyl*, Enduronyl Forte*, Harmonyl, Oreticyl Tab*
desipramine hydrochloride T: antidepressant, antianxiety agent P: dibenzazepine tricyclic antidepressant	Norpramin, Pertofran‡, Pertofrane
deslanoside (desacetyl-lanatoside C) T: antiarrhythmic, inotropic P: digitalis glycoside	Cedilanid†, Cedilanid-D
desmopressin acetate T: antidiuretic; hemostatic agent P: posterior pituitary hormone	DDAVP, Minirin‡, Stimate
desonide T: anti-inflammatory P: topical adrenocorticoid	DesOwen, Tridesilon
desoximetasone T: anti-inflammatory P: topical adrenocorticoid	Topicort
dexamethasone T: anti-inflammatory, immunosuppressant P: glucocorticoid	Aeroseb-Dex, Decaderm, Decadron, Decaspray*, Deronil, Dexasone†, Dexone, Hexadrol, Maxidex Ophthalmic Suspension, Maxitrol*, Mymethasone, NeoDecadron*, NeoDecaspray Aerosol*
dexamethasone acetate T: anti-inflammatory, immunosuppressant P: glucocorticoid	Dalalone D.P., Dalalone L.A., Decadron L.A., Decaject-L.A., Decameth L.A., Dexacen LA, Dexasone-LA, Dexone LA, Dexon LA, Solurex-LA
dexamethasone sodium phosphate T: anti-inflammatory, immunosuppressant P: glucocorticoid	Ak-Dex, Dalalone, Decadrol, Decadron Phosphate, Decadron Phosphate Ophthalmic, Decadron Phosphate Turbinaire, Decadron Phosphate with Xylocaine Injection*, Decaject, *(continued)*

---

† Available in Canada only.   ‡ Available in Australia only.   * Combination product.

GENERIC NAME AND CLASSIFICATIONS	TRADE NAMES
dexamethasone sodium phosphate *(continued)*	Decameth, Dex, Dexacen, Dexacidin*, Dexasone†, Dexon, Dexone, Hexadrol Phosphate, Maxidex Ophthalmic, NeoDecadron*, Neomycin Sulfate and Dexamethasone Sodium Phosphate Cream*, Neomycin Sulfate and Dexamethasone Sodium Phosphate Ophthalmic Solution*, Solurex
dexchlorpheniramine maleate T: antihistamine (H₁-receptor antagonist), antipruritic P: propylamine-derivative antihistamine	Dexchlor, Poladex TD, Polaramine, Polaramine Expectorant*, Polaramine Repetabs, Polargen
dextran, high molecular weight (dextran 70, dextran 75) T: plasma volume expander P: glucose polymer	Gentran 75, Macrodex
dextran, low molecular weight (dextran 40) T: plasma volume expander P: glucose polymer	Gentran 40, Rheomacrodex
dextranomer T: topical debriding agent P: synthetic polysaccharide	Debrisan, Envisan
dextroamphetamine sulfate T: central nervous system stimulant, short-term adjunctive anorexigenic agent, sympathomimetic amine P: amphetamine	Amodex*, Dexedrine, Dextrobar*, Ferndex, Oxydess II, Robese, Spancap #1, Trimex*
dextromethorphan hydrobromide T: antitussive (nonnarcotic) P: levorphanol derivative (dextrorotatory methyl ether)	Ambenyl-D*, Anti-Tuss DM*, Anti Tussive*, Balminil D.M., Bayer Cough Syrup for Children*, Benylin DM, Breachol*, Broncho-Grippol-DM†, Capahist-DMH*, CDM Expectorant*, Centuss*, Cerose-DM*, Cheracol-D*, Cheratussin*, Chexit*, Codimal DM*, Colrex Syrup*, Comtrex*, Conar*, Conar-A*, Congespirin for Children*, Contac Cough and Sore Throat Formula*, Contact Cough Formula*, Contac Jr. Children's Cold Medicine*, Contac Nighttime Cold Medicine*, Contac Severe Cold For-

T Therapeutic classification.   P Pharmacologic classification.

GENERIC NAME AND CLASSIFICATIONS	TRADE NAMES
dextromethorphan hydrobromide *(continued)*	mula Caplets*, Co-Tylenol*, Cremacoat 1, Delsym, Dimacol*, DM Cough, Donatussin Syrup*, Dorcol Children's Syrup*, Glycotuss-DM*, Guiatuss DM Syrup*, Halls Mentho-Lyptus Decongestant Cough Formula*, Hold, Hycoff-A Syrup*, Infantuss*, Koffex†, Mediquell, Neo-DM†, Nilcol*, Niltuss*, Novahistine DMX Liquid*, Nyquil*, Orthoxicaol*, Partuss*, Pediacare 1, Pertussin 8 Hour Cough Formula, Phenergran with Dextromethorphan*, Polytuss-DM*, Pyranistan Syrup*, Quelidrine Syrup*, Queltuss*, Rentuss*, Robidex†, Robitussin-CF*, Robitussin-DM*, Rondec-DM Oral Drops*, Rondec-DM Syrup*, Scotuf*, Scotuss*, Sedatuss†, Shertuss Liquid*, Silexin*, Sorbase Cough Syrup*, Spantuss*, Spec-T Sore Throat Cough Suppressant Lozengers*, St. Joseph for Children, Sucrets Cough Control Formula*, Synatuss-One*, Thor Syrup*, Tolu-Sed DM*, Tonecol*, Triamin*, Trind-DM Liquid*, Triaminicol Multi-Symptom Cold, Tusquelin-DM*, Tussagesic*, Tussaminic*, Tussar-DM*, Tussi-Organidin DM Liquid*, Unproco*, Vicks Children's Cough Syrup*, Vicks Cough Silencers*, Vicks Daycare*, Vicks Formula 44*, Waltussin DM*
dextrose (D-glucose) T: total parenteral nutrition component, caloric agent, fluid volume replacement P: carbohydrate	Aminosyn II with Dextrose*, Aminosyn II with Electrolytes in Dextrose*
dextrothyroxine sodium (d-thyroxine sodium) T: antilipemic P: thyroid hormone	Choloxin
dezocine T: analgesic P: opiate (narcotic) agonist-antagonist	Dalgan

---

GENERIC NAME AND CLASSIFICATIONS	TRADE NAMES
diazepam T: antianxiety agent; skeletal muscle relaxant; amnesic agent; anticonvulsant; sedative-hypnotic P: benzodiazepine	Apo-Diazepam†, Diazemuls†, Diazepam Intensol, E-Pam†, Meval†, Novodipam†, Q-Pam, Rival†, Valium, Valrelease, Vasepam, Vivol†, Zetran
diazoxide T: antihypertensive, antihypoglycemic P: peripheral vasodilator	Hyperstat
diazoxide, oral T: antihypertensive, antihypoglycemic P: peripheral vasodilator	Proglycem
dichlorphenamide T: antiglaucoma agent P: carbonic anhydrase inhibitor	Daranide
diclofenac sodium T: antiarthritic agent, anti-inflammatory P: nonsteroidal anti-inflammatory	Voltaren, Voltaren SR†
dicloxacillin sodium T: antibiotic P: penicillinase-resistant penicillin	Dycill, Dynapen, Pathocil
dicumarol (bishydroxycoumarin) T: oral anticoagulant P: coumarin derivative	
dicyclomine hydrochloride T: antimuscarinic, gastrointestinal antispasmodic P: anticholinergic	Antispas, Bemote, Bentyl, Bentylol†, Bentyl with Phenobarbital*, Byclomine, Dibent, Di-Cyclonex, Dilomine, Di-Spaz, Formulex†, Lomine†, Merbentyl‡, Neoquess Injection, Or-Tyl, Spasmoban†, Spasmoject, Tiactin*, Viscerol†
didanosine T: antiviral P: purine nucleoside	Videx
dienestrol (dienoestrol) T: topical estrogen P: estrogen	AVC/Dienestrol Cream*, DV, Ortho Dienestrol

---

T Therapeutic classification.   P Pharmacologic classification.

GENERIC NAME AND CLASSIFICATIONS	TRADE NAMES
diethylpropion hydro-chloride T: short-term adjunctive anorexigenic, sympathomimetic amine P: amphetamine	Nobesine†, Propion†, Tenuate, Tenuate Dospan, Tepanil, Tepanil Ten-Tab
diethylstilbestrol (stilboestrol) T: estrogen replacement, antineoplastic, postcoital contraceptive (unlabeled use) P: estrogen	DES, D.I.T.I. Creme*, Furacin-E Urethral Inserts*, Stilboestrol
diethylstilbestrol diphosphate T: estrogen replacement, antineoplastic, postcoital contraceptive (unlabeled use) P: estrogen	Honvol†, Stilphostrol
difenoxin hydrochloride T: antidiarrheal P: opioid agonist	Lyspafen‡, Motofen*
diflorasone diacetate T: anti-inflammatory P: topical adrenocorticoid	Florone, Flutone, Maxiflor, Psorcon
diflunisal T: nonnarcotic analgesic, antipyretic, anti-inflammatory agent P: nonsteroidal anti-inflammatory, salicyclic acid derivative	Dolobid
digitoxin T: antiarrhythmic agent, inotropic agent P: digitalis glycoside	Crystodigin, Foxalin*
digoxin T: antiarrhythmic, inotropic P: digitalis glycoside	Lanoxicaps, Lanoxin, Novodigoxin†
digoxin immune FAB (ovine) T: digitalis glycoside antidote P: antibody fragment	Digibind

---

† Available in Canada only.   ‡ Available in Australia only.   * Combination product.

GENERIC NAME AND CLASSIFICATIONS	TRADE NAMES
dihydroergotamine mesylate T: vasoconstrictor P: ergot alkaloid	D.H.E. 45, Dihydergot‡, Plexonal*
dihydrotachysterol T: antihypocalcemic P: vitamin D analog	AT-10‡, DHT, Hytakerol
dihydroxyaluminum sodium carbonate T: antacid P: aluminum salt	Rolaids
diltiazem hydrochloride T: antianginal P: calcium channel blocker	Cardizem, Cardizem SR
dimenhydrinate T: antihistamine (H_1-receptor antagonist), antiemetic and antivertigo agent P: ethanolamine-derivative antihistamine	Andrumin‡, Apo-Dimenhydrinate†, Calm X, Dimentabs, Dinate, Dommanate, Dramamine, Dramamine Chewable, Dramamine Liquid, Dramanate, Dramilin, Dramocen, Dramoject, Dymenate, Gravol†, Hydrate, Marmine, Motion-Aid, Nauseatol†, Novodimenate†, PMS-Dimenhydrinate†, Reidamine, Tega-Vert, Travamine†, Travs‡, Triptone Caplets, Wehamine
dimercaprol T: heavy metal antagonist P: chelating agent	BAL in Oil
dinoprostone (protoglandin E_2) T: oxytocic P: prostaglandin	Prostin E_2
diphenhydramine hydrochloride T: antihistamine (H_1-receptor antagonist), antiemetic and antivertigo agent, antitussive, sedative-hypnotic, topical anesthetic, antidyskinetic (anticholinergic) agent P: ethanolamine-derivative antihistamine	Allerdryl†, AllerMax, Ardebin*, Beldin, Belix, Bena-D, Bena-D 50, Benadryl, Benadryl Complete Allergy, Benahist 10, Benahist 50, Ben-Allergen-50, Benaphen, Bendylate*, Benoject-10, Benoject-50, Bentrac*, Benylin Cough, Benylin Dietetic†, Benylin Expectorant†, Benylin Pediatric†, Bydramine Cough, Compoz Diahist, Dihydrex, Diphenacen-50, Diphenadryl, Diphen Cough, Diphenhist, Dormarex 2, Eldadryl*, Fenylex*, Fenylhist, Fynex, Hydramine, Hydramyn, Hydril, Hyrexin-50,

---

T Therapeutic classification.   P Pharmacologic classification.

GENERIC NAME AND CLASSIFICATIONS	TRADE NAMES
diphenhydramine hydrochloride *(continued)*	Insomnal†, Nervine Nighttime Sleep-Aid, Noradryl, Nordryl, Nytol with DPH, Sleep-Eze 3, Sominex, Sominex Liquid, Symptrol*, Tusstat*, Twilite, Valdrene, Wehdryl, Ziradryl*
diphenidol hydrochloride T: antiemetic P: anticholinergic	Vontrol
diphenoxylate hydrochloride T: antidiarrheal P: opiate	Diaction*, Diphenatol, Lofene, Logen, Lomanate, Lomotil*, Lonox, Lo-Trol, Low-Quel, Nor-Mil
diphtheria and tetanus toxoids, adsorbed T: diphtheria and tetanus prophylaxis agent P: toxoid	
diphtheria and tetanus toxoids and pertussis vaccine (DPT) T: diphtheria, tetanus, and pertussis prophylaxis P: combination toxoid and vaccine	Tri-Immunol
diphtheria antitoxin, equine T: diphtheria antitoxin P: antitoxin	
dipivefrin T: antiglaucoma agent P: sympathomimetic agent	Propine
dipyridamole T: coronary vasodilator, platelet aggregation inhibitor P: pyrimidine analog	Apo-Dipyridamole†, Persantin 100‡, Persantine
disopyramide T: ventricular antiarrhythmic, supraventricular antiarrhythmic, atrial antitachyarrhythmic P: pyridine-derivative antiarrhythmic	Rythmodan†

GENERIC NAME AND CLASSIFICATIONS	TRADE NAMES
disopyramide phosphate T: ventricular antiarrhythmic, supraventricular antiarrhythmic, atrial antitachyarrhythmic P: pyridine-derivative antiarrhythmic	Napamide, Norpace, Norpace CR, Rythmodan LA†
disulfiram T: alcoholic deterrant P: aldehyde dehydrogenase inhibitor	Antabuse, Cronetal, Ro-Sulfiram-500
divalproex sodium T: anticonvulsant P: carboxylic acid derivative	Depakote, Epival†, Valcote‡
dobutamine hydrochloride T: inotropic agent P: adrenergic, beta$_1$ agonist	Dobutrex
docusate calcium (dioctyl calcium sulfosuccinate) T: emollient laxative P: surfactant	Pro-Cal-Sof, Surfak
docusate potassium (dioctyl potassium sulfosuccinate) T: emollient laxative P: surfactant	Dialose, Diocto-K, Kasof
docusate sodium (dioctyl sodium sulfosuccinate) T: emollient laxative P: surfactant	Afko-Lube, Barc*, Bevitone*, Calotabs*, Colace, Coloxyl‡, Coloxyl Enema Concentrate‡, Constiban*, Correctol*, Dialose Plus*, Diocto, Dioeze, Diolox*, Dio-Soft*, Diosuccin, Dio-Sul, Disanthrol*, Disolan*, Disonate, Di-Sosul, Di-Sosul Forte*, DOK-250, DOK Liquid, Doss 300, Doxinate, D-S-S, Dubbalax-B*, Dubbalax-N*, Duosol, Easy-Lax Plus*, Ex-Lax*, Feen-A-Mint*, Fer-Regules*, Ferro-Sequels*, Genasoft, Genericace*, Gentlax*, Geriplex-FS*, Hemaferrin*, Hemaspan*, Kapseal*, Laxadan*, Laxinate 100, Materna 1.6 Tabs*, Modane Soft, Neolax*, Neo-Vadrin D-D-S*, Nuvac*, Peri-Colace*, Peri-Pantyl*, Prosal*, Pro-Sof, Pro-Sof Liquid Concentrate, Pro-Sof 250, Recoup*, Rectalad Enema*, Regulax SS, Regutol, Rodox*, Sarolax*, Senokapp-DDS*, Senokot*,

GENERIC NAME AND CLASSIFICATIONS	TRADE NAMES
docusate sodium *(continued)*	Stulex, Tri-Vac*, Vagesic Plus Suppositories*
domperidone T: antiemetic P: dopamine antagonist	Motilium†‡
dopamine hydrochloride T: inotropic, vasopressor P: adrenergic	Intropin, Revimine†‡
doxacurium chloride T: skeletal muscle relaxant, adjunct in anesthesia P: neuromuscular blocking agent	Nuromax
doxapram hydrochloride T: central nervous system and respiratory stimulant P: analeptic	Dopram
doxazosin mesylate T: antihypertensive P: alpha-adrenergic blocking agent	Cardura
doxepin hydrochloride T: antidepressant P: tricyclic antidepressant	Adapin, Deptran‡, Sinequan, Triadapin†
doxorubicin hydrochloride T: antineoplastic P: antineoplastic antibiotic (cell cycle–phase nonspe- cific)	Adriamycin‡, Adriamycin PFS, Adriamycin RDF
doxycycline T: antibiotic P: tetracycline	Doxylin‡, Vibramycin
doxycycline hyclate T: antibacterial P: tetracycline	Doxy-Caps, Doxychel, Doxy-Lemmon, Doxy-Tabs, Doxy-100, Doxy-200, Vibramycin, Vibra-Tabs
doxycycline hydrochloride T: antibacterial P: tetracycline	Cyclidox‡, Doryx‡, Vibramycin‡, Vibramycin IV‡, Vibra-Tabs 50‡
dronabinol (tetrahydrocan- nabinol) T: antiemetic P: cannabinoid	Marinol

---

GENERIC NAME AND CLASSIFICATIONS	TRADE NAMES
droperidol T: tranquilizer P: butyrophenone derivative	Droleptan‡, Inapsine, Innovar*
dyclonine hydrochloride T: local anesthetic P: unclassified local anesthetic	Dyclone
dyphylline T: bronchodilator P: xanthine derivative	Bronkolate-G*, Brophylline, Dilin, Dilor, Dilor-G*, Dyflex, Dylline, Emfabid, Hycoff-A*, Lufyllin, Protophylline†

E

GENERIC NAME AND CLASSIFICATIONS	TRADE NAMES
echothiophate iodide (ecothiopate iodide) T: miotic P: cholinesterase inhibitor	Phospholine Iodide
econazole nitrate T: antifungal P: synthetic imidazole derivative	Ecostatin, Spectazole
edetate calcium disodium T: heavy metal antagonist P: chelating agent	Calcium Disodium Versenate, Calcium EDTA
edetate disodium T: heavy metal antagonist P: chelating agent	Allerest*, Dacriose*, Disodium EDTA, Disotate, Endrate, P.S.P. IV Injection*, Sinarest*, Solu-Pred*, Swim-Eye Drops*
edrophonium chloride T: cholinergic agonist, diagnostic agent P: cholinesterase inhibitor	Enlon, Reversol, Tensilon
eflornithine hydrochloride (DMFO) T: antiprotozoal P: ornithine decarboxylase inhibitor	Ornidyl
emetine hydrochloride T: amebicide P: ipecac alkaloid	Coryza*, Golacol*
enalaprilat T: antihypertensive P: angiotensin-converting enzyme inhibitor	Vasotec I.V.
enalapril maleate T: antihypertensive P: angiotensin-converting enzyme inhibitor	Amprace‡, Renitec‡, Vaseretic*, Vasotec
enoxacin T: antibiotic P: fluoroquinolone	Comprecin, Penetrex

---

† Available in Canada only.   ‡ Available in Australia only.   * Combination product.

GENERIC NAME AND CLASSIFICATIONS	TRADE NAMES
ephedrine hydrochloride T: bronchodilator, vasopressor, nasal decongestant P: adrenergic	Co-Xan*, Derma-Medicone-HC*, Fedrine†, Golacol*, Histacon*, KIE*, Lardet*, MediHaler-Iso*, Quadrinal*, Panaphyllin*, Quelidrine Syrup*, Tedral Elixir*, Tedral SA*, Theo-Span*, TSG Croup Liquid*
ephedrine sulfate T: bronchodilator, vasopressor, nasal decongestant P: adrenergic	Amphedrine*, Asma-Lief*, Asminorel*, BME*, Bronkaid Tabs*, Bronkolixir*, Bronkotabs*, Ceepa*, Co-Xan*, Derma Medicone*, Derma Medicone HC*, Ectasule*, Efedron Nasal Jelly, Enuretol*, Ephed II, Ephedrine and Nembutal-25*, Eponal*, Golacal*, Isi-Asminyl*, Isophed*, Kie*, Lardet*, Marax*, Marax DF*, Mudrane GG*, Mudrane Tablets*, Neogen*, Panaphyllin*, Pazo*, Pyrralan*, Quadrinal*, Quelidrine*, Quibron*, Rectacort*, Romaphed*, Tedral-25*, T-E-P Compound*, Theofedral*, Theofenal*, Thor Syrup*, Va-tro-nol Nose Drops, Wyanoids*, Wyanoids HC*
epinephrine T: bronchodilator, vasopressor, cardiac stimulant, local anesthetic (adjunct), topical antihemorrhagic, antiglaucoma agent P: adrenergic	Adrenalin, Ardecaine Injection*, Bronkaid Mist, Bronkaid Mistometer†, Dysne-Inhal†, Primatene Mist Solution
epinephrine bitartrate T: bronchodilator, vasopressor, cardiac stimulant, local anesthetic (adjunct), topical antihemorrhagic, antiglaucoma agent P: adrenergic	AsthmaHaler, Broniten Mist*, Bronkaid Mist Suspension*, Epitrate, Medihaler-Epi, Mytrate, Pilocarpine*, Primatene Mist Suspension
epinephrine hydrochloride T: bronchodilator, vasopressor, cardiac stimulant, local anesthetic (adjunct), topical antihemorrhagic, antiglaucoma agent P: adrenergic	Adrenalin Chloride, Epicar*, Epifrin, Epi-Pen, Epi-Pen Jr., Glaucon*, Sus-Phrine

T Therapeutic classification.   P Pharmacologic classification.

GENERIC NAME AND CLASSIFICATIONS	TRADE NAMES
epinephryl borate T: antiglaucoma agent P: ophthalmic sympathomimetic	Epinal, Eppy/N
epoetin alfa (erythropoietin) T: glycoprotein P: antianemic agent	Epogen, Procrit
ergonovine maleate (ergometrine maleate) T: oxytocic P: ergot alkaloid	Ergotrate Maleate
ergotamine tartrate T: vasoconstrictor P: ergot alkaloid	Bellergal*, Cafergot*, Cafergot P-B*, Ergkatal*, Ergomar, Ergostat, Ergotatropin*, Gynergen†, Medihaler-Ergotamine, Wigraine*
erythrityl tetranitrate T: antianginal, vasodilator P: nitrate	Cardilate, Cardilate-P*
erythromycin base T: antibiotic P: erythromycin	Apo-Erythro base†, EMU-V‡, E-Mycin, Eryc, Eryc Sprinkle, Ery-Tab, Erythromid†, Ilotycin, Novorythro†, PCE Dispersatabs, Robimycin
erythromycin estolate T: antibiotic P: erythromycin	Ilosone, Novorythro†
erythromycin ethylsuccinate T: antibiotic P: erythromycin	Apo-Erythro-ES†, E.E.S., E-Mycin E, EryPed, Erythrocin, Pediamycin, Wyamycin E
erythromycin gluceptate T: antibiotic P: erythromycin	Ilotycin
erythromycin lactobionate T: antibiotic P: erythromycin	Erythrocin
erythromycin stearate T: antibiotic P: erythromycin	Apo-Erythro-S†, Erypar, Erythrocin, Novorythro†, Wyamycin S
erythromycin (topical) T: antibiotic P: erythromycin	Akne-mycin, AS, Erycette, EryDerm, EryGel, Ery-Sol†, ETS†, Ilotycin Ophthalmic, Sans-Acne†, T-Stat†, Staticin

---

† Available in Canada only.   ‡ Available in Australia only.   * Combination product.

GENERIC NAME AND CLASSIFICATIONS	TRADE NAMES
esmolol hydrochloride T: antiarrhythmic P: beta$_1$-adrenergic blocking agent	Brevibloc
estazolam T: hypnotic P: benzodiazepine	ProSom
esterified estrogens T: estrogen replacement, antineoplastic P: estrogen	Estratab, Estromed†, Menest, Neo-Estrone†
estradiol (oestradiol) T: estrogen replacement, antineoplastic P: estrogen	Depo-Testadiol*, Estrace, Estrace Vaginal Cream, Estraderm, Estro Plus*, Hormonin*, Horm-Triad*, Sanestro*
estradiol cypionate T: estrogen replacement, antineoplastic P: estrogen	D-Diol*, depGynogen, Depo-Estradiol, Depo-Testadiol*, Dep-Tesestro*, Dep-Testradiol*, Duo-Cyp*, Duracrine*, Dura-Estrin, E-Cypionate, Estran-C*, Estro-Cyp, Estrofem, Estroject-L.A., Estronol-LA, Menoject L.A.*, Span F.M.*, T.E. Lonate P.A.*
estradiol valerate (oestradiol valerate) T: estrogen replacement, antineoplastic P: estrogen	Ardiol*, Deladumone*, Delatestadiol*, Delestrogen, Depo-testadiol*, Dioval, Ditate DS*, Duoval-P.A.*, Duragen 10, Duragen 20, Duragen 40, Estate*, Estradiol L.A., Estra-Testrin*, Estraval, Estraval P.A., Estra-L 20, Estra-L 40, Feminate, Femogex, Gynogen L.A., Hy-Gestradol*, Hylutin-Est*, L.A.E., Menaval, Primogyn Depot‡, Repose E-40*, Repose-TE*, Retadiamone*, Ru-Est-Span 20, Ru-Est-Span 40, Span-Est-Test 4*, Teev*, Tesogen*, Testanate*, Valergen 10, Valergen 20, Valergen 40, Valertest*
estramustine phosphate sodium T: antineoplastic P: estrogen, alkylating agent	Emcyt, Estracyst
estrogens, conjugated T: estrogen replacement, antineoplastic, antiosteoporotic P: estrogen	C.E.S.†, Conjugated Estrogens C.S.D.†, Estritone*, Estrogenic Mixture Preparations*, Estrogenic Substance Preparations*, Milprem*, Ovlin*, Premarin, Premarin Intrave-

T Therapeutic classification.   P Pharmacologic classification.

GENERIC NAME AND CLASSIFICATIONS	TRADE NAMES
estrogens, conjugated *(continued)*	nous, Premarin with Methyltesto-sterone*, Progens
estrone (oestrone) T: estrogen replacment P: estrogen	Andesterone*, Android-G*, An-drone*, Anestro*, Angen*, Di-Hormone Suppositories*, Di-Met*, Diorapin*, Dl-Steroid *, Duovin-S*, Dura-Keelin*, Estratest*, Estrogenic Mixture Preparations*, Estrogenic Substance Preparations*, Estrone Aqueous, Estrone "5", Estronol, Estro-Plus*, Estrovag*, Estro-V HC*, Geramine*, Geratic Forte*, Geria-mic*, Geritag*, Hormonin*, Kestrone, Mer-Estrone*, Ovest*, Ovulin*, Pro-estrone*, Sanestro*, Sodestrin*, Spanestrin-P*, Tesogen*, Testrone*, Theelin Aqueous, Tostestro*, Tri-Or-apin*, Tripole-F*
estropipate (piperazine es-trone sulfate) T: estrogen replacment P: estrogen	Ogen
ethacrynate sodium T: diuretic P: loop diuretic	Edecrin Sodium
ethacrynic acid T: diuretic P: loop diuretic	Edecril‡, Edecrin
ethambutol hydrochloride T: antitubercular agent P: semisynthetic antitubercular	Etibi†, Myambutol
ethaverine hydrochloride T: peripheral vasodilator P: isoquinoline derivative	Ethaquin, Ethatab, Ethavex-100, Isovex
ethchlorvynol T: sedative-hypnotic P: chlorinated tertiary acetylenic carbinol	Placidyl
ethinyl estradiol (ethinyloestradiol) T: estrogen replacement, anti-neoplastic P: estrogen	Brevicon*, Demulen*, Estinyl, Feminone, Halodrin*, Loestrin 1/20*, Loestrin 1.5/30*, Lo/Ovral*, Modicon 21*, Modicon 28*, Nordette*, Norinyl*, Norlestrin*, Norlestrin Fe*, Ortho-Novum 1/35*, Ortho-Novum *(continued)*

GENERIC NAME AND CLASSIFICATIONS	TRADE NAMES
ethinyl estradiol *(continued)*	7/7/7*, Ortho-Novum 10/11*, Ovalin*, Ovcon*, Ovral*, Triphasil*
ethinyl estradiol and ethynodiol diacetate T: contraceptive P: estrogen and progestin combination	*monophasic:* Demulen 1/35, Demulen 1/50
ethinyl estradiol and levonorgestrel T: contraceptive P: estrogen and progestin combination	*monophasic:* Levlen, Nordette *triphasic:* Tri-Levlen, Triphasil
ethinyl estradiol and nor-ethindrone T: contraceptive P: estrogen and progestin combination	*monophasic:* Brevicon, Genora 0.5/35, Genora 1/35, Modicon, N.E.E. 1/35, Nelova 0.5/35 E, Nelova 1/35 E, Norcept-E 1/35, Norethin 1/35 E, Norinyl 1+35, Ortho-Novum 1/35, Ovcon-35, Ovcon-50 *biphasic:* Nelova 10/11, Ortho Novum 10/11 *triphasic:* Ortho Novum 7/7/7, Tri-Norinyl
ethinyl estradiol and nor-ethindrone acetate T: contraceptive P: estrogen and progestin combination	*monophasic:* Loestrin 21 1/20, Loestrin 21 1.5/30, Norlestrin 21 1/50, Norlestrin 21 2.5/50
ethinyl estradiol and norgestrel T: contraceptive P: estrogen and progestin combination	*monophasic:* Lo/Ovral, Ovral
ethinyl estradiol, norethin-drone acetate, and ferrous fumarate T: contraceptive with iron P: estrogen, progestin, and iron combination	*monophasic:* Loestrin Fe 1/20, Loestrin Fe 1.5/30, Norlestrin Fe 1/50, Norlestrin Fe 2.5/50
ethionamide T: antitubercular agent P: isonicotinic acid derivative	Trecator-SC
ethosuximide T: anticonvulsant P: succinimide derivative	Zarontin

---

T Therapeutic classification.　　　P Pharmacologic classification.

GENERIC NAME AND CLASSIFICATIONS	TRADE NAMES
ethotoin T: anticonvulsant P: hydantoin derivative	Peganone
ethylestrenol (ethyloestrenol) T: antianemic, anti-osteoporotic, antiarthritic P: anabolic steroid	Maxibolin, Orabolin‡
ethylnorepinephrine hydro-chloride T: bronchodilator P: adrenergic agonist	Bronkephrine
etidocaine hydrochloride T: local anesthetic, amide P: sodium channel blocker	Duranest
etidronate disodium T: antihypercalcemic P: pyrophosphate analog	Didronel
etodolac T: antiarthritic P: nonsteroidal anti-inflammatory	Lodine
etomidate T: I.V. anesthetic, sedative P: nonbarbiturate hypnotic	Amidate, Hypnomidate
etoposide (VP-16) T: antineoplastic P: podophyllotoxin (cell cycle–phase specific, G_2 and late S phases)	VePesid
etretinate T: antipsoriatic agent P: retinoid	Tegison
eye irrigation solutions T: ophthalmic cleansing solution P: isotonic solution for ophthalmic use	Blinx, Collyrium, Dacriose, Eye-Stream, I-Lite Eye Drops, Lauro Eye Wash, Lavoptik Eye Wash, Murine Eye Drops, Neo-Flo, Sterile Normal Saline (0.9%)

F

GENERIC NAME AND CLASSIFICATIONS	TRADE NAMES
factor IX complex T: systemic hemostatic P: blood derivative	Konyne-HT, Profilnine Heat-Treated, Proplex T
famotidine T: antiulcer agent P: histamine$_2$-receptor antagonist	Pepcid, Pepcidine‡
fat emulsions T: parenteral nutrition support P: lipid	Intralipid 10%, Intralipid 20%, Liposyn 10%, Liposyn 20%, Liposyn II 10%, Liposyn II 20%, Soyacal 10%, Soyacal 20%, Travamulsion 10%, Travamulsion 20%
felodipine T: antihypertensive P: calcium channel antagonist	Plendil
fenfluramine hydrochloride T: short-term adjunctive anorexigenic agent, indirect-acting sympathomimetic amine P: amphetamine congener	Ponderal†, Ponderal Pacaps†, Ponderax‡, Ponderax Pacaps‡, Pondimin, Pondimin Extentabs
fenoprofen calcium T: nonnarcotic analgesic, antipyretic, anti-inflammatory P: nonsteroidal anti-inflammatory	Nalfon
fentanyl citrate T: analgesic, adjunct to anesthesia, anesthetic P: opioid agonist	Sublimaze
fentanyl citrate with droperidol T: analgesic, general anesthetic P: opiod agonist	Innovar
fentanyl transdermal system T: analgesic P: opioid agonist	Duragesic-25, Duragesic-50, Duragesic-75, Duragesic-100

T Therapeutic classification.   P Pharmacologic classification.

GENERIC NAME AND CLASSIFICATIONS	TRADE NAMES
ferrous fumarate T: hematinic P: oral iron supplement	Bevitone*, C-Ron*, C-Ron F.A.*, Cytoferin*, Eldofe, Eldofe-C*, Feostat, Ferancee*, Ferancee HP*, Ferranol, Fer-Regules*, Ferropyl Chewable Tabs*, Ferro-Sequels*, Fersamal†, Fumasorb, Fumerin, Hemaspan*, Hemocyte, Ircon, Mani-ron, Minhema Chewable Tabs*, Norinyl-L Fe 28*, Norlestrin Fe*, Novofumar†, Ortho-Novum 1/50*, Ortho-Novum 1/80*, Palafer†, Span-FF
ferrous gluconate T: hematinic P: oral iron supplement	Fergon, Ferralet, Fertinic†, Hemocr-ine*, I.L.X. with B₁₂*, Novoferro-gluc†, Pergrava #2*, Simron*, Stuart Hematinic*
ferrous sulfate T: hematinic P: oral iron supplement	Feosol, Fer-In-Sol, Feritard‡, Fermalox*, Fero-Folic-500*, Fero-Grad†, Fero-Grad-500*, Fero-Gradumet, Ferolix, Ferospace, Ferralyn, Fespan‡, Folvron*, Hemo-crine*, Intrin*, Irospan, Mol-Iron, Mol-Iron with Vitamin C*, Novoferro-sulfa†, Slow-Fe, Telefon
fibrinolysin and desoxyribonuclease T: topical debriding agent P: proteolytic enzyme	Elase
filgrastim (granulocyte colony stimulating factor; G-CSF) T: colony stimulating factor P: biological response modifier	Neupogen
flavoxate hydrochloride T: urinary tract spasmolytic P: flavone derivative	Urispas
flecainide acetate T: ventricular antiarrhythmic P: benzamide derivative, local anesthetic (amide)	Tambocor
floxuridine T: antineoplastic P: antimetabolite (cell cycle–phase specific, S phase)	FUDR

GENERIC NAME AND CLASSIFICATIONS	TRADE NAMES
fluconazole T: antifungal P: bis-triazole derivative	Diflucan
flucytosine (5-FC) T: antifungal P: fluorinated pyrimidine	Ancobon
fludarabine phosphate T: antileukemic P: antimetabolite	Fludara
fludrocortisone acetate T: mineralocorticoid replacement therapy P: mineralocorticoid, glucocorticoid	Florinef
flumazenil T: antidote P: benzodiazepine antagonist	Mazicon
flunisolide T: anti-inflammatory, anti-asthmatic P: glucocorticoid	AeroBid Inhaler, Nasalide, Rhinalar Nasal Mist‡
fluocinolone acetonide T: anti-inflammatory P: topical adrenocorticoid	Fluocet, Fluonid, Flurosyn, Neomycin and Fluocinolone Acetonide Cream*, Neo-Synalar*, Synalar, Synemol
fluocinonide T: anti-inflammatory P: topical adrenocorticoid	Lidemol†, Lidex, Lidex-E, Topsyn
fluorescein sodium T: diagnostic aid P: dye	Fluorescite, Fluor-I-Strip, Fluor-I-Strip A.T., Ful-Glo, Funduscein Injections
fluorometholone T: ophthalmic anti-inflammatory P: corticosteroid	FML Liquifilm Ophthalmic, FML S.O.P., Neo-Oxylone*
fluorouracil (5-fluorouracil; 5-FU) T: antineoplastic P: antimetabolite (cell cycle–phase specific, S phase)	Adrucil, Efudex, Fluoroplex
fluoxetine T: antidepressant P: serotonin uptake inhibitor	Prozac

T Therapeutic classification.   P Pharmacologic classification.

GENERIC NAME AND CLASSIFICATIONS	TRADE NAMES
fluoxymesterone T: androgen replacement, antineoplastic P: androgen	Android F, Halodrin*, Halotestin, Ora-Testryl
fluphenazine decanoate T: antipsychotic P: phenothiazine (piperazine derivative)	Modecate Decanoate‡, Prolixin Decanoate
fluphenazine enanthate T: antipsychotic P: phenothiazine (piperazine derivative)	Moditen Enanthate†, Prolixin Enanthate
fluphenazine hydrochloride T: antipsychotic P: phenothiazine (piperazine derivative)	Anatensol‡, Apo-Fluphenazine†, Moditen HCl†, Moditen HCl-HP†, Permitil, Prolixin
flurandrenolide T: anti-inflammatory P: topical adrenocorticoid	Cordran, Cordran-N*, Cordran SP, Cordran Tape, Drenison†, Drenison 1/4†, Drenison Tape†, Neomycin Sulfate and Flurandrenolide*
flurazepam hydrochloride T: sedative-hypnotic P: benzodiazepine	Apo-Flurazepam†, Dalmane, Durapam, Novoflupam†, Sam-Pam†
flurbiprofen T: antiarthritic P: nonsteroidal anti-inflammatory, phenylalkanoic acid derivative	Ansaid
flurbiprofen sodium T: ophthalmic anti-inflammatory, antimiotic P: nonsteroidal anti-inflammatory	Ocufen
flutamide T: antineoplastic agent P: nonsteroidal antiandrogen	Eulexin
fluticasone propionate T: topical anti-inflammatory P: corticosteroid	Cutivate
foscarnet T: antiviral P: pyrophosphate analog	Foscavir

---

† Available in Canada only.   ‡ Available in Australia only.   * Combination product.

GENERIC NAME AND CLASSIFICATIONS	TRADE NAMES
fosinopril sodium T: antihypertensive P: angiotensin-converting enzyme inhibitor	Monopril
fructose (levulose) T: parenteral nutritional therapy, caloric agent P: carbohydrate	
furazolidone T: antibacterial, antiprotozoal agent P: nitrofuran derivative	Furoxone
furosemide (frusemide) T: diuretic, antihypertensive P: loop diuretic	Apo-Furosemide†, Furomide M.D., Furoside†, Lasix, Lasix Special†, Myrosemide, Novosemide†, Urex‡, Urex-M‡, Uritol†
furazolidone T: antibacterial, antiprotozoal agent P: nitrofuran derivative	Furoxone
furosemide (frusemide) T: diuretic, antihypertensive P: loop diuretic	Apo-Furosemide†, Furomide M.D., Furoside†, Lasix, Lasix Special†, Myrosemide, Novosemide†, Urex‡, Urex M‡, Uritol†

G

GENERIC NAME AND CLASSIFICATIONS

TRADE NAMES

gallamine triethiodide
T: skeletal muscle relaxant
P: nondepolarizing neuromuscular blocking agent

Flaxedil

gallium nitrate
T: antihypercalcemic agent
P: heavy metal

Ganite

ganciclovir (DHPG)
T: antiviral agent
P: synthetic nucleoside

Cytovene

gemfibrozil
T: antilipemic
P: fibric acid derivative

Lopid

gentamicin
T: antibiotic
P: aminoglycoside

Gentacidin

gentamicin sulfate
T: antibiotic
P: aminoglycoside

Cidomycin‡, Garamycin, Garamycin Ophthalmic Solution*, Genoptic, Gentafair, Jenamicin

gentian violet (methylrosaniline chloride; crystal violet)
T: topical antibacterial, anti-fungal
P: triphenylmethane (rosaniline) dye

Genapax, Hyva*

glipizide
T: antidiabetic agent
P: sulfonylurea

Glucotrol, Minidiab‡

glucagon
T: antihypoglycemic, diag-nostic agent
P: antihypoglycemic agent

glutethimide
T: sedative-hypnotic
P: piperidinedione

Doriden, Doriglute

GENERIC NAME AND CLASSIFICATIONS	TRADE NAMES
glyburide T: antidiabetic agent P: sulfonylurea	DiaBeta, Euglucon†, Micronase
glycerin T: laxative (osmotic), ophthalmic osmotic agent, adjunctive agent in treating glaucoma, lubricant P: trihydric alcohol, ophthalmic osmotic vehicle	Cortisporin Otic Solution Sterile*, Fleet Babylax, Kerid Ear Drops*, Rectalad*, Sani-Supp, Vioform-HC*
glycerin, anhydrous T: ophthalmic osmotic agent, adjunctive agent in treating glaucoma P: trihydric alcohol, ophthalmic osmotic vehicle	Ophthalgan
glycopyrrolate T: antimuscarinic, gastrointestinal antispasmodic P: anticholinergic	Robinul, Robinul Forte
gold sodium thiomalate T: antiarthritic P: gold salt	Myochrisine
gonadorelin acetate T: fertility agent P: gonadotropin-releasing hormone	Lutrepulse
gonadorelin hydrochloride T: diagnostic agent P: luteinizing hormone-releasing hormone	Factrel
gonadotropin, chorionic (HCG) T: spermatogenesis stimulant P: gonadotropin	Antuitrin, A.P.L., Chorex, Follutein, Glukor*, Pregnyl, Profasi HP
goserelin acetate T: luteinizing hormone-releasing hormone analog P: synthetic decapeptide	Zoladex
griseofulvin microsize T: antifungal P: *Penicillium* antibiotic	Fulcin‡, Fulvicin-U/F, Grifulvin V, Grisactin, Grisovin‡, Grisovin 500‡, Grisovin-FP

T Therapeutic classification.   P Pharmacologic classification.

GENERIC NAME AND CLASSIFICATIONS	TRADE NAMES
griseofulvin ultramicrosize T: antifungal P: *Penicillium* antibiotic	Fulvicin P/G, Grisactin Ultra, Griseostatin‡, Gris-PEG
guaifenesin (glyceryl guaiacolate) T: expectorant P: propanediol derivative	Actifed-C Syrup*, Ambenyl-D*, Anti-Tuss, Anti-Tuss DM*, Asbron G*, Balminil Expectorant†, Baytussin, Breonesin, Bronchovent*, Brondecon*, Bronkaid*, Bronkolate-G*, Bronkolixir*, Bronkotabs*, Bro-Tane Expectorant*, Bur-Tuss*, CDM-Expectorant*, Cheracol-D*, Colrex Expectorant, Comtrex Cough Formula*, Conar-A*, Congestac*, Contac*, Cortane*, Co-Xan*, Cremacoat 2, Dilaudid*, Dilor-G*, Dimacol*, Donatussin*, Dorcol Children's Cough Syrup*, Emagrin Forte*, Embron*, Emfaseem*, Entex*, Fedahist*, Gee-Gee, GG-CEN, Glyate, Glycotuss, Glycotuss-DM*, Glynaphen*, Glytuss, Guiatuss, Guiatuss DAC Syrup*, Guiatuss DM Syrup*, Guiatussin with Codeine*, Guistrey Fortis*, Halotussin, Humibid L.A., Hycoff-A Syrup*, Hycotuss Expectorant*, Hytuss, Hytuss-2X, Isoclor Expectorant*, Kleer*, Lanatuss*, Lardet Expectorant*, Malotuss, Mudrane GG-2*, Naldecon Senior EX, Neo-Spec†, Neothylline GG-Liquid*, Nilcol*, Nortussin, Novahistine DMX Liquid*, Novahistine Expectorant*, Panaphyllin*, Partuss-A*, Phenatuss*, PMP Expectorant*, Polaramine Expectorant*, Polyectin*, Polytuss-DM*, Pyranistan*, Queltuss*, Quibron*, Quibron Plus*, Quibron-300*, Rentuss*, Resyl†, Robafen, Robitussin, Robitussin AC*, Robitussin CF*, Robitussin DAC*, Robitussin DM*, Robitussin PE*, Rymed*, Rymed TR*, Santussin*, Scotuf*, Scotuss*, Silexin*, Slo-Phyllin GG*, Sorbase Cough Syrup*, S-T Expectorant, Sudafed Cough Syrup*, Synatuss-One*, Synophylate-GG*, Theocolate*, Thor Syrup*, Tolu-Sed*, Tolu-Sed DM*, Tonecol Cough Syrup*, Triaminic Expectorant*, Triaminic Expecto- *(continued)*

GENERIC NAME AND CLASSIFICATIONS	TRADE NAMES
guaifenesin (*continued*)	rant with Codeine*, Trihistin Expectorant*, Tussafed Expectorant*, Tussar-SF*, Tussar-2*, Unproco*, Vicks Children's Cough Syrup*, Vicks Daycare*, Vicks Formula 44*, Waltussin*
guanabenz acetate T: antihypertensive P: centrally acting antiadrenergic agent	Wytensin
guanadrel sulfate T: antihypertensive P: adrenergic neuron blocking agent	Hylorel
guanethidine sulfate T: antihypertensive P: adrenergic neuron blocking agent	Apo-Guanethidine†, Esimil*, Ismelin
guanfacine hydrochloride T: antihypertensive P: centrally acting antiadrenergic	Tenex

H

GENERIC NAME AND CLASSIFICATIONS	TRADE NAMES
Haemophilus b conjugate vaccine, diphtheria CRM$_{197}$ protein conjugate (HbOC) T: bacterial vaccine P: vaccine	HibTITER
Haemophilus b conjugate vaccine, diphtheria toxoid conjugate (PRP-D) T: bacterial vaccine P: vaccine	ProHIBIT
Haemophilus b conjugate vaccine, meningococcal protein conjugate (PRP-OMP) T: bacterial vaccine P: vaccine	PedvaxHIB
Haemophilus b polysaccharide vaccine T: bacterial vaccine P: vaccine	b-CapsaI, Hib-Imune
halazepam T: antianxiety agent P: benzodiazepine	Paxipam
halcinonide T: anti-inflammatory P: topical adrenocorticoid	Halciderm, Halog
halobetasol propionate T: topical anti-inflammatory P: corticosteroid	Ultravate
haloperidol T: antipsychotic P: butyrophenone	Apo-Haloperidol†, Haldol, Halperon, Novoperidol, Peridol†, Serenace‡
haloperidol decanoate T: antipsychotic P: butyrophenone	Haldol Decanoate, Haldol LA†
haloperidol lactate T: antipsychotic P: butyrophenone	Haldol

---

† Available in Canada only.　　‡ Available in Australia only.　　* Combination product.

GENERIC NAME AND CLASSIFICATIONS	TRADE NAMES
haloprogin T: topical antifungal P: synthetic antifungal	Halotex
heparin calcium T: anticoagulant P: anticoagulant	Calcilean†, Calciparine, Caprin, Uni-parin-Ca‡
heparin sodium T: anticoagulant P: anticoagulant	Hepalean†, Heparin Lock Flush Solution (Tubex), Hep Lock, Liquaemin Sodium, Uniparin‡
hepatitis B immune globulin, human T: hepatitis B prophylaxis product P: immune serum	H-BIG, Hep-B-Gammagee, HyperHep
hepatitis B vaccine, plasma derived T: viral vaccine P: vaccine	Heptavax-B
hepatitis B vaccine, recombinant T: viral vaccine P: vaccine	Engerix-B, Recombivax HB
hetastarch T: plasma volume expander P: amylopectin derivative	Hespan
hexocyclium methylsulfate T: antimuscarinic, gastrointestinal antispasmodic P: anticholinergic	Tral Filmtabs
histoplasmin T: skin test antigen P: *Histoplasma capsulatum*	Histolyn-CYL
histrelin acetate T: treatment of precocious puberty P: gonadotropin-releasing hormone agonist	Supprelin
homatropine hydrobromide T: cycloplegic, mydriatic P: anticholinergic agent	Diaquel*, Homatrine, Homatropine, Isopto Homatropine

---

T Therapeutic classification.   P Pharmacologic classification.

GENERIC NAME AND CLASSIFICATIONS	TRADE NAMES
hyaluronidase T: adjunctive agent to increase absorption and dispersion of injected drugs P: protein enzyme	Wydase
hydralazine hydrochloride T: antihypertensive P: peripheral vasodilator	Alazine, Apresazide *, Apresoline, Apresoline-Esidrix Tablets*, Dralserp*, Harbolin*, Hydralazide*, Hydroserpine Plus*, Novo-Hylazin†, Ser-Ap-Es*, Serapine*, Serpasil-Apresoline*, Supres‡, Thia-Serpa-Zine*, Unipres*
hydrochlorothiazide T: diuretic, antihypertensive P: thiazide diuretic	Aldactazide*, Aldoril*, Apo-Hydro†, Apresazide*, Apresoline-Esidrix Tablets*, Aquapres-R*, Dichlotride‡, Diuchlor H†, Dyazide*, Esidrix, Esimil*, Harbolin*, Hydralazide*, HydroDIURIL, Hydropres*, Hydroserp*, Hydroserpine*, Hydrotensin-50*, Hyperserp*, Inderide*, Mallopress*, Mictrin, Moduretic*, Natrimax†, Novohydrazide†, Oretic, Oreticyl*, Ser-Ap-Es*, Serapine*, Serpasil-Esidrix Tablets*, Thia-Serp-25*, Thia-Serp-50*, Thiuretic, Timolide*, Trandate*, Unipres*, Urozide†, Vaseretic*
hydrocortisone T: adrenocorticoid replacement, anti-inflammatory P: glucocorticoid, mineralocorticoid	Aerseb-HC, Aticort, Aural Acute*, Bafil*, Biotic Ophthalmic with Hydrocortisone Ointment*, Biscolan HC*, Caquin*, Carmol HC*, Cetacort, Coracin*, Cor-Oticin*, Cort-Dome, Cortef, Cortenema, Corticoid*, Cortin*, Cortisporin Cream*, Cortisporin Ointment*, Cortisporin Ophthalmic Ointment*, Cortisporin Ophthalmic Suspension*, Cortisporin Otic Solution Sterile*, Cortisporin Otic Suspension*, Cortnal, Cortizone-5, Cortril, Cremesone, Delacort, Dermapax*, Dermarex*, DermiCort, Dermolate, Doctient-HC*, Drotic Sterile Otic Solution*, Durel-Cort, Ecosone, HC Cream, HC-Form*, HI-Cor-2.5, HIL-20 Lotion*, Hycort†, Hycortone, Hydrelt*, Hydrocort*, Hydrocortex, Hydrocortone, Hysone*, Hytone, Ivocort, Kencort*, Lanvisone*, Lorox- *(continued)*

GENERIC NAME AND CLASSIFICATIONS	TRADE NAMES
hydrocortisone *(continued)*	ide-HC Lotion*, Maso-Cort, Microcort, Neo-Cort*, Neocortef Cream*, Nutracort, Opthocort*, Orabase HCA, Oto*, Otobiotic*, Otocalm-H Ear Drops*, Otoreid-HC*, Otostan HC*, Penecort, Proctocort, Pyocidin-Otic*, Racet LCD*, Rhus Tox HC, Rocort, Sherform-HC*, Squibb-HC‡, Stera-Form*, Tar-Quin-HC*, Terra-Cortil*, Unicort, Vanox-ide-HC*, V-Cort*, Vioform-HC*
hydrocortisone acetate T: adrenocorticoid replacement, anti-inflammatory P: glucocorticoid, mineralocorticoid	Anusol HC*, Biosone, Biscolan HC*, Carmol HC*, Chloromycetin-HC Ophthalmic*, Coly-Mycin-S Otic*, Cortaid, Cortamed†, Cortef Acetate*, Corticaine*, Corticreme†, Cortifoam, Dermacort‡, Dermacort Ointment‡, Derma-Medicone-HC*, Epifoam, Epiform*, Furacin*, Hydrocortone Acetate, Komed*, Lidaform-HC*, Lida-Mantle HC*, Mantadil*, Mycort Lotion, Neo-Cortef*, Neo-Polycin-HC Ointment*, Ophthocort*, Proctofoam*, Proctofoam-HC, Rectacort*, Viotag Cream*, Wyanoids HC*
hydrocortisone cypionate T: adrenocorticoid replacement P: glucocorticoid, mineralocorticoid	Cortef
hydrocortisone sodium phosphate T: adrenocorticoid replacement P: glucocorticoid, mineralocorticoid	Hydrocortone Phosphate
hydrocortisone sodium succinate T: adrenocorticoid replacement P: glucocorticoid, mineralocorticoid	A-HydroCort, Solu-Cortef
hydrocortisone valerate T: anti-inflammatory P: glucocorticoid	Westcort Cream

---

T Therapeutic classification.   P Pharmacologic classification.

GENERIC NAME AND CLASSIFICATIONS	TRADE NAMES
hydroflumethiazide T: diuretic, antihypertensive P: thiazide diuretic	Diucardin, Saluron, Salutensin*, Salutensin-Demi*
hydromorphone hydro-chloride T: analgesic, antitussive P: opioid	Dilaudid, Dilaudid HP, Dilocol
hydroxychloroquine sulfate T: antimalarial, anti-inflam-matory agent P: 4-aminoquinoline	Plaquenil
hydroxyprogesterone caproate T: progestin, antineoplastic P: progestin	Delalutin†, Duralutin, Gesterol L.A., Hy-Gestadol*, Hy-Gesterone, Hylutin, Hylutin-Est*, Hyprogest, Hyproval P.A., Hyroxon, Pro-Depo, Prodrox
hydroxyurea T: antineoplastic P: antimetabolite (cell cycle–phase specific, S phase)	Hydrea
hydroxyzine hydrochloride (hydroxyzine embonate) T: antianxiety agent; seda-tive; antipruritic; antiemetic; antispasmodic P: antihistamine (piperazine derivative)	Anxanil, Apo-Hydroxyzine†, Atarax, Atozine, Durrax, Enarax*, E-Vista, Hydroxacen, Hyzine-50, Marax*, Marax DF Syrup*, Multipax†, Novohydroxyzin†, Quiess, Vistacon, Vistaject, Vistaquel, Vistaril, Vistazine
hydroxyzine pamoate T: antianxiety agent; seda-tive; antipruritic; antiemetic; antispasmodic P: antihistamine (piperazine derivative)	Hy-Pam, Vamate, Vistaril
hyoscyamine T: anticholinergic P: belladonna alkaloid	Cystospaz
hyoscyamine sulfate T: anticholingergic P: belladonna alkaloid	Anaspaz, Aridol*, Azo-Cyst*, Barbeloid*, Brobelaa-P.B.*, Butabell HMB*, Cystospaz, Cystospaz-M, Cys-tospaz-SR*, Detal*, Donnacin*, Donnatal*, Donnatal #2*, Donnazyme*, Eldonal*, Enterex*, Fenatron*, Haponal*, Hyonal*, Hytrona*, Kapigam*, Kinesed*, Levsin, Levsinex Timecaps, Mass- *(continued)*

GENERIC NAME AND CLASSIFICATIONS	TRADE NAMES
hyoscyamine sulfate *(continued)*	Donna*, Neoquess, Nilspasm*, Palsorb Improved*, Peece Kaps*, Phenahist-TR*, Scopine*, Sedamine*, Sedapar*, Setamine*, Spabelin Elixir*, Spasaid*, Spasmolin*, Spasquid*, Stannitol*, Ultabs*, Uriprel*

GENERIC NAME AND CLASSIFICATIONS	TRADE NAMES
ibuprofen T: nonnarcotic analgesic, antipyretic, anti-inflammatory P: nonsteroidal anti-inflammatory	Aches-N-Pain, Advil, Amersol†, Apo-Ibuprofen†, Brufen‡, Cap-Profen, Genpril, Haltran, Ibuprin, Inflam‡, Medipren Caplets, Medipren Tablets, Midol-200, Motrin, Motrin IB, Novoprofen†, Nuprin, Pamprin-IB, Rafen‡, Rufen, Trendar
idarubicin T: antineoplastic P: antibiotic antineoplastic	Idamycin
idoxuridine (IDU) T: antiviral agent P: halogenated pyrimidine	Herplex, Stoxil
ifosfamide T: antineoplastic P: alkylating agent (cell cycle–phase nonspecific)	Ifex
imipenem-cilastatin sodium T: antibiotic P: carbapenem (thienamycin class); beta-lactam antibiotic	Primaxin*
imipramine hydrochloride T: antidepressant P: dibenzazepine tricyclic antidepressant	Apo-Imipramine†, Imiprin‡, Impril†, Janimine, Novo-Pramine†, Tofranil, Tripramine
imipramine pamoate T: antidepressant P: dibenzazepine tricyclic antidepressant	Tofranil-PM
immune globulin intramuscular (IGIM; IG; gamma globulin) T: immune serum P: immune serum	Gamastan, Gammar, Immunoglobin
immune globulin intravenous (IGIV) T: immune serum P: immune serum	Gamimine N, Gammagard, Sandoglobulin, Venoglobulin-I

GENERIC NAME AND CLASSIFICATIONS	TRADE NAMES
indapamide T: diuretic, antihypertensive P: thiazide-like diuretic	Lozide†, Lozol, Natrilix†
indecainide hydrochloride T: antiarrhythmic (class IC) P: sodium channel blocking agent	Decabid
indomethacin T: nonnarcotic analgesic, antipyretic, anti-inflammatory P: nonsteroidal anti-inflammatory	Apo-Indomethacin†, Arthrexin†, Indameth, Indocid†‡, Indocid SR†, Indocin, Indocin SR, Indomed, Novomethacin†, Rheumacin‡, Zendole
indomethacin sodium trihydrate T: nonnarcotic analgesic, antipyretic, anti-inflammatory P: nonsteroidal anti-inflammatory	Apo-Indomethacin†, Indocid†, Indocin I.V., Indometh, Novomethacin
influenza virus vaccine, 1991-1992 trivalent types A & B (purified surface antigen) T: viral vaccine P: vaccine	Flu-Imune
influenza virus vaccine, 1991-1992 trivalent types A & B (subvirion or split virion) T: viral vaccine P: vaccine	Fluogen Split, Fluzone Split, Influenza Virus Vaccine (Split)
influenza virus vaccine, 1991-1992 trivalent types A & B (whole virion) T: viral vaccine P: vaccine	Fluzone (Whole)
insulin injection (regular insulin, crystalline zinc insulin) T: antidiabetic agent P: pancreatic hormone	Actrapid HM‡, Actrapid HM Penfill‡, Actrapid MC‡, Actrapid MC Penfill‡, Beef Regular Iletin II, Humulin R, Hypurin Neutral‡, Insulin 2‡, Novolin R, Novolin R Penfill, Pork Regular Iletin II, Regular (Concentrated) Iletin II, Regular Iletin I, Regular Purified Pork Insulin, Velosulin, Velosulin Human‡, Velosulin Insuject

---

T Therapeutic classification.   P Pharmacologic classification.

GENERIC NAME AND CLASSIFICATIONS	TRADE NAMES
insulin zinc suspension, prompt (semilente) T: antidiabetic agent P: pancreatic hormone	Semilente Iletin I, Semilente Insulin, Semilente MC Pork‡, Semilente Purified Pork
insulin zinc suspension (lente) T: antidiabetic agent P: pancreatic hormone	Humulin L, Lente Iletin I, Lente Iletine II, Lente Insulin, Lente MC‡, Lente Purified Pork Insulin, Monotard HM‡, Monotard MC‡, Novolin L
insulin zinc suspension, extended (ultralente) T: antidiabetic agent P: pancreatic hormone	Ultralente Iletin I, Ultralente Insulin, Ultralente Purified Beef, Ultratard HM‡, Ultratard MC‡
interferon alfa-2a, recombinant (rIFN-A) T: antineoplastic P: biological response modifier	Roferon-A
interferon alfa-2b recombinant (IFN-alpha 2) T: antineoplastic P: biological response modifier	Intron A
interferon alfa-n3 T: antineoplastic P: biological response modifier	Alferon N
interferon gamma-1b T: antineoplastic P: biological response modifier	Actimmune
intravascular perfluorochemical emulsion T: oxygen-carrying solution P: perfluorochemical emulsion	Fluosol
invert sugar T: nonelectrolyte fluid replacement, fluid volume expander, caloric agent P: carbohydrate	Travert
iodinated glycerol T: expectorant P: organic iodine complex	Iophen Elixir, Myodine, Organidin, R-Ger Elixir

---

† Available in Canada only.　　‡ Available in Australia only.　　* Combination product.

GENERIC NAME AND CLASSIFICATIONS	TRADE NAMES
iodochlorhydroxyquin (clioquinol) T: topical antibacterial, topical antifungal P: halogenated 8-hydroxyquinoline	Bafil Lotion*, Caquin*, Cortin*, Dermarex Cream*, Enterex*, Hc-Form*, HIL-20 Lotion*, Hydrelt*, Hydrocort*, Hysone*, Kencort*, Lanvisone*, Lidaform-HC*, Nystaform*, 1+1-Creme*, Racet LCD*, Sherform-HC*, Stera-Form*, Tar-Quin-HC*, Torofor, V-Cort*, Vioform, Viotag*
iodoquinol (diiodohydroxyquin) T: amebicide P: iodinated 8-hydroxyquinoline	Diodoquin†, Moebiquin, Yodoxin
ipecac syrup T: emetic P: alkaloid emetic	Histapco*, Pectoral*, Polyectin*, Proclan Expectorant with Codeine*, Proclan VC Expectorant with Codeine*, Quelidrine*
ipratropium bromide T: bronchodilator P: anticholinergic	Atrovent
iron dextran T: hematinic P: parenteral iron supplement	Hydextran, Imferon, K-FeRON
isocarboxazid T: antidepressant P: monoamine oxidase inhibitor	Marplan
isoetharine hydrochloride T: bronchodilator P: adrenergic	Arm-a-Med Isoetharine, Beta-2, Bisorine, Bronkosol, Dey-Dose Isoetharine, Dey-Dose Isoetharine S/F, Dey-Lute Isoetharine, Dispos-a-Med Isoetharine
isoetharine mesylate T: bronchodilator P: adrenergic	Bronkometer
isoflurophate T: antiglaucoma agent P: miotic, cholinesterase inhibitor	Floropryl

GENERIC NAME AND CLASSIFICATIONS	TRADE NAMES
isoniazid (INH) T: antitubercular agent P: isonicotinic acid hydrazine	Calpas-INAH-6*, Calpas-INH*, Calpas Isoxine*, DOW-Isoniazid, Isotamine†, Laniazid, Niadox*, Nydrazid, Pasna Tri-Pack*, P-I-N Forte*, PMS-Isoniazid†, Rimactane*, Teebaconin*, Triniad Plus 30*, Uniad-Plus*
isophane insulin suspension (neutral protamine Hagedorn insulin, NPH) T: antidiabetic agent P: pancreatic hormone	Beef NPH Iletin II, Humulin N, Humulin NPH‡, Hypurin Isophane‡, Insulatard‡, Insulatard Human‡, Insulatard NPH, Isotard MC‡, Novolin N, NPH Iletin I, NPH Insulin, NPH Purified Pork, Pork NPH Iletin II, Protaphane HM‡, Protaphane HM Penfill‡, Protaphane MC‡
isophane insulin suspension with insulin injection T: antidiabetic agent P: pancreatic hormone	Actraphane HM‡, Actraphane HM Penfill‡, Actraphane MC‡, Mixtard, Mixtard Human‡, Novolin 70/30
isopropamide iodide T: muscarinic, gastrointestinal antispasmodic P: anticholinergic	Darbid, Iso-Perazine*, Tyrimide‡
isoproterenol T: bronchodilator, cardiac stimulant P: adrenergic	Aerolone, Dey-Dose Isoproterenol, Dispos-a-Med Isoproterenol, Isuprel, MediHaler-Iso*, Vapo-Iso
isoproterenol hydrochloride T: bronchodilator, cardiac stimulant P: adrenergic	Aerolone Compound*, Asminorel*, Duo-MediHaler*, Iso-Asminyl*, Isophed*, Isuprel, Isuprel Mistometer, Norisodrine Aerotrol
isoproterenol sulfate T: bronchodilator, cardiac stimulant P: adrenergic	Medihaler-Iso, Norisodrine*
isosorbide T: antiglaucoma agent P: osmotic diuretic	Ismotic
isosorbide dinitrate T: antianginal agent, vasodilator P: nitrate	Apo-ISDN†, Cedocard-SR†, Coronex†, Dilatrate-SR, Iso-Bid, Isonate, Isorbid, Isordil, Isotrate, Nitro-Spray‡, Novosorbide†, Sorbitrate, Sorbitrate SA, Sorbitrate with Phenobarbital*

GENERIC NAME AND CLASSIFICATIONS	TRADE NAMES
isosorbide mononitrate T: antianginal P: nitrate	ISMO
isotretinoin T: antiacne agent, keratiniza- tion stabilizer P: retinoic acid derivative	Accutane, Roaccutane‡
isoxsuprine hydrochloride T: peripheral vasodilator P: beta-adrenergic agonist	Duvadilan‡, Vasodilan, Vasoprine
isradipine T: antihypertensive P: calcium channel blocker	DynaCirc

JKL

GENERIC NAME AND CLASSIFICATIONS	TRADE NAMES
kanamycin sulfate T: antibiotic P: aminoglycoside	Kanasig‡, Kantrex, Klebcil
kaolin and pectin mixtures T: antidiarrheal P: adsorbent	B-K-P Mixture*, Cholactabs*, Diastay*, Donnagel-MB†, Duosorb*, Kao-Con†, Kaoparin*, Kaopectate, Kaopectate Concentrate, Kao-tin, Kapectin*, Kapectolin, Ka-Pek with Paregoric*, Kapigam*, Kapinal*, Kay-Pec*, KBP/O*, K-P, K-Pek, Metropectin*, Palsorb Improved*, Parepectolin*, Pectocel*, Pectocomp*, Pecto-Kalin*, Wescola Antidiarrheal Stomach Upset*
ketamine hydrochloride T: intravenous anesthetic P: dissociative anesthetic	Ketalar
ketoconazole T: antifungal P: imidazole derivative	Nizoral
ketoprofen T: nonnarcotic analgesic, antipyretic, anti-inflammatory P: nonsteroidal anti-inflammatory	Orudis, Orudis E†, Orudis SR†‡
ketorolac tromethamine T: analgesic P: nonsteroidal anti-inflammatory	Toradol
ketotifen fumarate T: antiasthmatic P: antihistamine	Zaditen
labetalol hydrochloride T: antihypertensive P: alpha- and beta-adrenergic blocking agent	Normodyne, Presolol‡, Trandate, Trandate HCT*
lactulose T: laxative P: disaccharide	Cephulac, Cholac, Chronulac, Constilac, Duphalac, Enulose, Lactulax†

---

† Available in Canada only.   ‡ Available in Australia only.   * Combination product.

GENERIC NAME AND CLASSIFICATIONS	TRADE NAMES
leucovorin calcium (citrovorum factor or folinic acid) T: vitamin, antidote P: folic acid derivative	Wellcovorin
leuprolide acetate T: antineoplasic P: gonadotropic hormone	Lucrin‡, Lupron, Lupron Depot
levamisole hydrochloride T: antineoplastic P: immunomodulator	Ergamisol
levobunolol hydrochloride T: antiglaucoma agent P: beta-adrenergic blocking agent	Betagan
levocarnitine (L-carnitine) T: nutritional supplement P: amino acid derivative	Carnitor, Vitacarn
levodopa (L-dopa) T: antiparkinsonian agent P: precursor of dopamine	Dopar, Larodopa, Levopa, Parda, Rio-Dopa, Sinemet*
levonorgestrel T: contraceptive P: progestin	Nordette*, Norplant System, Triphasil*
levorotatory alkaloids of belladonna T: antiulcer agent, treatment of hypermotility P: indirect-acting parasympathomimetic	Bellafoline
levorphanol tartrate T: analgesic, adjunct to anesthesia P: opioid	Levo-Dromoran
levothyroxine sodium (T_4 or L-thyroxine sodium) T: thyroid hormone replacement agent P: thyroid hormone	Eltroxin†, Levoid, Levothroid, Levoxine, Oroxine‡, Synthroid*, Synthrox, Thyrolar*
lidocaine hydrochloride (lignocaine hydrochloride) T: ventricular antiarrhythmic, local anesthetic P: amide derivative	Aerosept*, Ardecaine*, Bafil*, Caine-2, Dalcaine, Decadron Phosphate with Xylocaine*, Dilocaine, Duo-Trach Kit, HIL-20 Lotion*, Kip First Aid Preps*, L-Caine-E*, Lidaform-HC*,

---

T Therapeutic classification.   P Pharmacologic classification.

GENERIC NAME AND CLASSIFICATIONS	TRADE NAMES
lidocaine hydrochloride (*continued*)	Lida-Mantle HC*, Lidoject-2, Lido Pen Auto-Injector, Lidosporin*, Medi-Quik*, Nervocaine 2%, Octocaine, Unguentine Spray*, Unguentine Plus*, Xylocaine, Xylocard‡
lincomycin hydrochloride T: antibiotic P: lincosamide	Lincocin
lindane T: scabicide, pediculicide P: chlorinated hydrocarbon insecticide	gBh†, Kwell, Kwellada†, Scabene
liothyronine sodium (T$_3$) T: thyroid hormone replacement agent P: thyroid hormone	Cyronine, Cytomel, Tertroxin‡
liotrix T: thyroid hormone replacement agent P: thyroid hormone	Euthroid, Thyrolar
lisinopril T: antihypertensive P: angiotensin-converting enzyme inhibitor	Prinivil, Zestril
lithium carbonate T: antimanic, antipsychotic P: alkali metal	Camcolit‡, Carbolith†, Duralith†, Eskalith, Eskalith CR, Lithane, Lithicarb‡, Lithizine†, Lithobid, Lithonate, Lithotabs, Priadel‡
lithium citrate T: antimanic, antipsychotic P: alkali metal	Cibalith-S
lomustine (CCNU) T: antineoplastic P: alkylating agent, nitrosourea (cell cycle–phase nonspecific)	CeeNU
loperamide T: antidiarrheal P: piperadine derivative	Imodium, Imodium A-D
loracarbef T: antibiotic P: carbacephem derivative	Lorabid

† Available in Canada only.   ‡ Available in Australia only.   * Combination product.

loratidine
T: nonsedating antihistamine
P: selective histamine₁-
antagonist

Claritin

lorazepam
T: antianxiety agent; seda-
tive-hypnotic
P: benzodiazepine

Alzapam, Apo-Lorazepam, Ativan,
Loraz, Novolorazem†

lovastatin
T: cholesterol-lowering agent
P: lactone

Mevacor

loxapine hydrochloride
T: antipsychotic
P: dibenzoxazepine

Loxapac†, Loxitane C, Loxitane I.M.

loxapine succinate
T: antipsychotic
P: dibenzoxazepine

Loxapac†, Loxitane

**lymphocyte immune globu-
lin (antithymocyte globulin
[equine] ATG)**
T: immunosuppressive agent
P: immunoglobulin

Atgam

lypressin
T: antidiuretic hormone
P: posterior pituitary hormone

Diapid

T Therapeutic classification.   P Pharmacologic classification.

M

GENERIC NAME AND CLASSIFICATIONS	TRADE NAMES
mafenide acetate T: topical antibacterial P: synthetic anti-infective	Sulfamylon
magaldrate (aluminum-magnesium complex) T: antiulcer agent P: antacid	Antiflux†, Lowsium, Riopan
magnesium carbonate T: antacid P: magnesium salt	Algicon*, Alkets*, Bufferin*, Bufferin Arthritis Strength*, Bufferin Arthritis Strength Tri-Buff*, Bufferin Extra Strength*, Di-Gel*, Escot*, Estomul M Liquid*, Eugel*, Glycogel*, Marablen*, Triactin*
magnesium chloride T: electrolyte replacement P: magnesium salt	Slow-Mag
magnesium citrate (citrate of magnesia) T: laxative P: magnesium salt	Citroma, Citro-Nesia
magnesium hydroxide T: antacid, antiulcer agent, laxative P: magnesium salt	Alsorb Gel*, Aludrox*, Ascripten*, Ascripten AD*, Ascripten Extra Strength*, Calciphen*, Cama*, Delcid*, Di-Gel*, Fermalox*, Gas-Eze*, Gelusil*, Kolantyl*, Laxsil*, Maalox*, Maalox Plus*, Magnatril*, Magnesia Magma, Milk of Magnesia, Mylanta*, Mylanta II*, Neutralox*, Nutrameg*, Silian Gel*, Simeco*, Simethox*, Triactin*, Trialka*, Vanquis*, Wingel*
magnesium oxide T: antacid P: magnesium salt	Alkets*, Buffaprin*, Bufferin Arthritis Strength Tri-Buff*, Bufferin Extra Strength*, Buffinol*, Cama Arthritis Strength*, Elekap*, Magnox*, Mag-Ox 400, Maox, Par-Mag, Uro-Mag
magnesium salicylate T: nonnarcotic analgesic, antipyretic, anti-inflammatory P: salicylate	Extra-Strength Doan's, Magan, Mobidin, Mobigesic*, Original Doan's

---

† Available in Canada only.   ‡ Available in Australia only.   * Combination product.

GENERIC NAME AND CLASSIFICATIONS	TRADE NAMES
magnesium sulfate T: anticonvulsant P: mineral, electrolyte	Vicon-C*, Vicon Forte*, Vicon Plus*
magnesium sulfate (epsom salts) T: laxative P: magnesium salt	
magnesium trisilicate T: antacid P: magnesium oxide and silicon dioxide	Antacid G*, Arcodex Antacid*, Azolid-A*, Butazolidin Alicia*, Escot*, Eulcin*, Gacid*, Gaviscon*, Kaosil*, Magnatril*, Malcogel*, Malcotabs*, Manalum*, Marblen*, Marcaid-2*, Silmagel*, Triactin*, Trisogel*, Trisomin
mannitol T: diuretic, prevention and management of acute renal failure or oliguria, reduction of intraocular or intracranial pressure, treatment of drug intoxication P: osmotic diuretic	Cystosal*, Cytal*, Gas-Eze*, Osmitrol†, Synthroid*
maprotiline hydrochloride T: antidepressant P: tricyclic antidepressant	Ludiomil
mazindol T: anorexigenic agent P: imidazole-isoindol	Mazanor, Sanorex
measles, mumps, and rubella virus vaccine, live T: viral vaccine P: vaccine	Lirutin*, M-M-RII
measles (rubeola) and rubella virus vaccine, live attenuated T: viral vaccine P: vaccine	Lirubel*, M-R-Vax II
measles (rubeola) virus vaccine, live attenuated T: viral vaccine P: vaccine	Attenuvax, M-M-R*, M-R-Vax*
mebendazole T: anthelmintic P: benzimidazole	Vermox

T Therapeutic classification.   P Pharmacologic classification.

GENERIC NAME AND CLASSIFICATIONS	TRADE NAMES
mecamylamine hydro-chloride T: antihypertensive P: ganglionic blocking agent	Inversine
mechlorethamine hydro-chloride (nitrogen mustard) T: antineoplastic P: alkylating agent (cell cycle–phase nonspecific)	Mustargen
meclizine hydrochloride (meclozine hydrochloride) T: antiemetic and antivertigo agent P: piperazine-derivative antihistamine	Ancolan‡, Antivert, Antivert/25, Antivert/50, Bonamine, Bonine, Dizmiss, Meni-D, Ru-Vert M
meclofenamate T: nonnarcotic analgesic, antipyretic, anti-inflammatory P: nonsteroidal anti-inflammatory	Meclomen
medium-chain triglycerides T: enteral nutrition therapy P: modular supplement	M.C.T.
medroxyprogesterone acetate T: progestin, antineoplastic P: progestin	Amen, Curretab, Cycrin, Depo-Provera, Provera
medrysone T: ophthalmic anti-inflammatory P: corticosteroid	HMS Liquifilm Ophthalmic
mefenamic acid T: nonnarcotic analgesic, antipyretic, anti-inflammatory P: nonsteroidal anti-inflammatory	Ponstan†, Ponstel
mefloquine hydrochloride T: antimalarial P: quinine derivative	Lariam
megestrol acetate T: antineoplastic P: progestin	Megace, Megostat‡

---

† Available in Canada only.   ‡ Available in Australia only.   * Combination product.

GENERIC NAME AND CLASSIFICATIONS	TRADE NAMES
melphalan (L-phenylala-nine mustard) T: antineoplastic P: alkylating agent (cell cycle–phase nonspecific)	Alkeran
meningitis vaccine T: bacterial vaccine P: vaccine	Menomune-A/C, Menomune-A/C/Y/W-135
menotropins T: ovulation stimulant, spermatogenesis stimulant P: gonadotropin	Pergonal
mepenzolate bromide T: antimuscarinic, gastrointestinal antispasmodic P: anticholinergic	Cantil, Cantil with Phenobarbital*
meperidine hydrochloride (pethidine hydrochloride) T: analgesic, adjunct to anesthesia P: opioid	Demerol, Demerol APAP*, Mepergan*
mephentermine sulfate T: vasopressor P: adrenergic	Wyamine
mephenytoin T: anticonvulsant P: hydantoin derivative	Mesantoin
mephobarbital T: anticonvulsant, nonspecific central nervous system depressant P: barbiturate	Koly-Tabs*, Mebaral, Tranquil*
mepivacaine hydrochloride T: local anesthetic P: amide local anesthetic	Carbocaine, Cavacaine, Isocaine
meprobamate T: antianxiety agent P: carbamate	Apo-Meprobamate†, Deprol*, Equagesic*, Equanil, Meditran, Meprospan, Milpath*, Milprem*, Miltrate*, Miltown, Neuramate, Novo-Mepro†, Pathibamate*, PMB 200*, Robam-Petn*, Sedabamate, Tranmep

GENERIC NAME AND CLASSIFICATIONS	TRADE NAMES
mercaptopurine (6-MP, 6-mercaptopurine) T: antineoplastic P: antimetabolite (cell cycle–phase specific, S phase)	Purinethol
mesalamine T: anti-inflammatory P: salicylate	Rowasa
mesna T: uroprotectant P: thiol derivative	Mesnex
mesoridazine besylate T: antipsychotic P: phenothiazine (piperidine derivative)	Serentil
mestranol and norethin-drone T: contraceptive P: estrogen and progestin combination	*monophasic:* Genora 1/50, Nelova 1/50 M, Norethin 1/50 M, Norinyl 1+50, Ortho-Novum 1/50
metaproterenol sulfate T: bronchodilator P: adrenergic	Alupent, Arm-A-Med Metaproterenol, Dey-Dose Metaproterenol, Dey-Med Metaproterenol, Metaprel
metaraminol bitartrate T: vasopressor P: adrenergic	Aramine
metaxalone T: skeletal muscle relaxant P: oxazolidinone derivative	
metformin T: oral hypoglycemic P: dimethybiguanide hydro-chloride	Glucophage†
methadone hydrochloride T: analgesic, narcotic detoxi-fication adjunct P: opioid	Dolophine, Methadose, Nodalin*, Physeptone‡
methamphetamine hydro-chloride T: central nervous system stimulant, short-term adjunc-tive anorexigenic, sympatho-mimetic amine P: amphetamine	Aridol*, Desoxyn, Desoxyn Gradumet, Fetamin*, Obe-Slim*, Span-RD*

---

† Available in Canada only.   ‡ Available in Australia only.   * Combination product.

GENERIC NAME AND CLASSIFICATIONS	TRADE NAMES
methantheline bromide T: antimuscarinic, gastrointestinal antispasmodic P: anticholinergic	Banthine, Banthine with Phenobarbital*
methazolamide T: adjunctive treatment for open-angle glaucoma, perioperatively for acute angle-closure glaucoma P: carbonic anhydrase inhibitor	Neptazane
methdilazine hydrochloride T: antihistamine (H_1-receptor antagonist), antipruritic P: phenothiazine derivative	Dilosyn†, Tacaryl
methenamine hippurate T: urinary tract antiseptic P: formaldehyde pro-drug	Hiprex, Hip-Rex†, Urex
methenamine mandelate T: urinary tract antiseptic P: formaldehyde pro-drug	Mandameth, Mandelamine, Sterine†, Thiacide*, Uriseamine*
methicillin sodium T: antibiotic P: penicillinase-resistant penicillin	Metin‡, Staphcillin
methimazole T: antihyperthyroid agent P: thyroid hormone antagonist	Tapazole
methocarbamol T: skeletal muscle relaxant P: carbonate derivative of guaifenesin	Delaxin, Marbaxin-750, Robaxin, Robomol-500, Robomol-750
methohexital sodium (methohexitone sodium) T: intravenous anesthetic P: barbiturate	Brevital Sodium, Brietal Sodium†‡
methotrexate T: antineoplastic P: antimetabolite (cell cycle–phase specific, S phase)	

GENERIC NAME AND CLASSIFICATIONS	TRADE NAMES
methotrexate sodium T: antineoplastic P: antimetabolite (cell cycle–phase specific, S phase)	Folex, Mexate, Rheumatrex
methotrimeprazine hydrochloride (levomepromazine hydrochloride) T: sedative, analgesic agent, antipruritic P: propylamino phenothiazine	Levoprome, Nozinan†
methoxsalen T: pigmenting, antipsoriatic agent P: psoralen derivative	Oxsoralen, Oxsoralen-Ultra
methscopolamine bromide T: antimuscarinic, gastrointestinal antispasmodic P: anticholinergic	Bobid*, Eulcin*, Pamine, Pamine PB*, Scoline-Amobarbital*, Symptrol*, Synt-PB*
methsuximide T: anticonvulsant P: succinimide derivative	Celontin
methyclothiazide T: diuretic, antihypertensive P: thiazide diuretic	Aquatensen, Duretic†, Enduron, Enduron M‡
methylcellulose T: bulk-forming laxative P: adsorbent	Canfield Lubricating Jelly*, Chloromycetin-HC Ophthalmic*, Citucel, Cologel, Efricel ⅛%*, Enterex*, Ex-Caloric*, Isopto Carbachol Solution*, Isopto Cetapred*, Isopto P-ES*, Lacril Artificial Tears*, Pepto-Bismal*, Rite-Diet*, Triactin*, Vernacel*
methyldopa T: antihypertensive P: centrally acting antiadrenergic agent	Aldoclor*, Aldomet, Aldomet M‡, Aldoril*, Apo-Methyldopa†, Dopamet†, Hydopa‡, Novomedopa†
methyldopate hydrochloride T: antihypertensive P: centrally acting antiadrenergic agent	Aldomet, Aldomet Ester Injection‡

† Available in Canada only.   ‡ Available in Australia only.   * Combination product.

GENERIC NAME AND CLASSIFICATIONS	TRADE NAMES
methylene blue T: urinary tract antiseptic, cyanide poisoning antidote, treatment of methemo-globinemia P: thiazine dye	Cystrea*, Hexalol*, Lanased*, Uriprel*, Urised*, Urolene Blue
methylergonovine maleate T: oxytocic P: ergot alkaloid	Methergine
methylphenidate hydro-chloride T: central nervous system stimulant (analeptic) P: piperidine central nervous system stimulant	Ritalin, Ritalin SR
methylprednisolone T: anti-inflammatory, im-munosuppressant P: glucocorticoid	Medrol†, Meprolone, Neo-Medrol Ointment*, Solu-Medrol*
methylprednisolone acetate T: anti-inflammatory, im-munosuppressant P: adrenocorticoid, gluco-corticoid	depMedalone, Depoject, Depo-Medrol, Depopred, Depo-Predate, D-Med, Duralone, Durameth, Medra-lone, Medrol Enpak, Medrone, Methylone, M-Prednisol, Neomycin Sulfate and Methylprednisolone Ace-tate Cream*, Neomedral*, Rep-Pred
methylprednisolone sodium succinate T: anti-inflammatory, im-munosuppressant P: glucocorticoid	A-Metha-pred, Medrol, Solu-Medrol
methyltestosterone T: androgen replacement P: androgen	Android, Estritone*, Metandren, Metandren Linguets, Oreton Methyl, Premarin with Methyltestosterone*, Testomet‡, Testred, Virilon*
methyprylon T: sedative-hypnotic P: piperidine-dione derivative	Noludar
methysergide maleate T: vasoconstrictor P: ergot alkaloid	Deseril‡, Sansert
metipranol T: antiglaucoma agent P: beta-adrenergic blocking agent	OptiPranol

GENERIC NAME AND CLASSIFICATIONS	TRADE NAMES
metoclopramide hydro-chloride T: antiemetic, gastrointestinal stimulant P: para-aminobenzoic acid (PABA) derivative	Maxeran†, Maxolon‡, Maxolon High Dose‡, Regla
metocurine iodide T: skeletal muscle relaxant P: nondepolarizing neuromuscular blocking agent	Metubine
metolazone T: diuretic, antihypertensive P: quinazoline derivative (thiazide-like) diuretic	Diulo, Mykrox, Zaroxolyn
metoprolol tartrate T: antihypertensive, adjunctive treatment of acute myocardial infarction P: beta-adrenergic blocking agent	Apo-Metoprolol†, Betaloc‡, Betaloc Durules†, Lopresor†, Lopresor SR†, Lopressor, Novometoprol†
metronidazole T: antibacterial, antiprotozoal, amebicide P: nitroimidazole	Apo-Metronidazole†, Flagyl, Metizol, Metrogyl‡, Metrozine‡, Metryl, Neo-Metric†, Novonidazol†, PMS Metronidazole†, Protostat
metronidazole (topical) T: antiprotozoal, antibacterial P: nitroimidazole	MetroGel
metronidazole hydro-chloride T: antibacterial, antiprotozoal, amebicide P: nitroimidazole	Flagyl I.V., Flagyl I.V. RTU, Metro I.V., Novonidazol†
metyrosine T: antihypertensive P: tyrosine hydroxylase inhibitor	Demser
mexiletine hydrochloride T: ventricular antiarrhythmic P: lidocaine analogue, sodium channel antagonist	Mexitil

GENERIC NAME AND CLASSIFICATIONS	TRADE NAMES
mezlocillin sodium T: antibiotic P: extended-spectrum penicillin, acyclamino-penicillin	Mezlin
miconazole T: antifungal P: imidazole derivative	Monistat I.V.
miconazole nitrate T: antifungal P: imidazole derivative	Micatin, Monistat-Derm Cream and Lotion, Monistat 7 Vaginal Cream, Monistat 7 Vaginal Suppository, Monistat 3 Vaginal Suppository
microfibrillar collagen hemostat T: hemostatic agent P: collagen derivative	Avitene
midazolam hydrochloride T: sedative, amnesic agent P: benzodiazepine	Versed
mineral oil (liquid petrolatum) T: laxative P: lubricant oil	Agoral Plain, Fleet Mineral Oil, Kondremul Plain, Liqui-Doss, Milkinol, Neo-Cultol, Zymenol
minocycline hydrochloride T: antibiotic P: tetracycline	Minocin, Minomycin‡, Minomycin IV‡
minoxidil T: antihypertensive P: peripheral vasodilator	Loniten, Minodyl
minoxidil (topical) T: hair-growth stimulant P: direct acting vasodilator	Rogaine
misoprostol T: antiulcer agent, gastric mucosal protectant P: prostaglandin E_1 analog	Cytotec
mitomycin (mitomycin-C) T: antineoplastic P: antineoplastic antibiotic (cell cycle–phase nonspecific)	Mutamycin

---

T Therapeutic classification.   P Pharmacologic classification.

GENERIC NAME AND CLASSIFICATIONS	TRADE NAMES
mitotane T: antineoplastic, antiadrenal agent P: chlorophenothane (DDT) analog	Lysodren
mitoxantrone hydro-chloride T: antineoplastic P: antibiotic antineoplastic	Novantrone
mivacurium T: neuromuscular blocking agent P: nicotinic cholinergic agonist	Mivacron
molindone hydrochloride T: antipsychotic P: dihydroindolone	Moban
mometasone furoate T: topical anti-inflammatory P: synthetic corticosteroid	Elocon
monooctanoin T: cholelitholytic P: esterified glycerol	Moctanin
moricizine hydrochloride T: antiarrhythmic P: sodium channel blocker	Ethmozine
morphine hydrochloride T: narcotic analgesic P: opioid	Morphitec†, M.O.S.†, M.O.S.-S.R.†
morphine sulfate T: narcotic analgesic P: opioid	Astramorph, Astramorph P.F., Duramorph PF, Epimorph†, Morphine H.P.†, MS Contin, MSIR, Pectoral Preps*, RMS Uniserts, Roxanol, Roxanol SR, Statex†
moxalactam disodium (latamoxef disodium) T: antibiotic P: third-generation cephalosporin	Moxalactam‡, Moxam
mumps skin test antigen T: skin test antigen P: viral antigen	MSTA

---

† Available in Canada only.   ‡ Available in Australia only.   * Combination product.

GENERIC NAME AND CLASSIFICATIONS	TRADE NAMES
mumps virus vaccine, live T: viral vaccine P: vaccine	Mumpsvax
mupirocin (pseudomonic acid A) T: topical anesthetic P: antibiotic	Bactroban
muromonab-CD3 T: immunosuppressive agent P: monoclonal antibody	Orthoclone OKT3

N

GENERIC NAME AND CLASSIFICATIONS	TRADE NAMES
nabumetone T: antiarthritic, anti-inflammatory P: nonsteroidal anti-inflammatory	Relafen
nadolol T: antihypertensive, antianginal P: beta-adrenergic blocking agent	Corgard
nafarelin acetate T: gonadotropin-releasing hormone analog P: synthetic decapeptide	Synarel
nafcillin sodium T: antibiotic P: penicillinase-resistant penicillin	Nafcil, Nallpen, Unipen
naftifine T: antifungal P: synthetic allylamine	Naftin
nalbuphine hydrochloride T: analgesic, adjunct to anesthesia P: narcotic agonist-antagonist; opioid partial agonist	Nubain
nalidixic acid T: urinary tract antiseptic P: quinolone antibiotic	NegGram
naloxone hydrochloride T: narcotic antagonist P: narcotic (opioid) antagonist	Narcan
naltrexone hydrochloride T: narcotic detoxification adjunct P: narcotic (opioid) antagonist	Trexan

GENERIC NAME AND CLASSIFICATIONS	TRADE NAMES
nandrolone decanoate T: erythropoietic agent, anabolic, antineoplastic P: anabolic steroid	Anabolin LA, Androlone-D, Deca-Durabolin, Decolone, Hybolin Decanoate, Kabolin, Nandrobolic L.A., Neo-Durabolic
nandrolone phenpropionate T: antineoplastic P: anabolic steroid	Anabolin IM, Androlone, Durabolin, Hybolin Improved, Nandrobolic
naphazoline hydrochloride T: decongestant, vasoconstrictor P: sympathomimetic agent	AK-Con, Albalon-A Liquifilm*, Albalon Liquifilm, Alkalon Ophthalmic Solution*, Alkalon Liquifilm Ophthalmic Solution*, Allerest, Clear Eyes, Degest 2, Estivin II, 4-Way Nasal Spray*, Naphcon, Naphcon A*, Naphcon Forte, Optazine‡, Privine, Vapocyn II Nasal Spray*, Vasoclear, Vasocon-A Ophthalmic Solution*, Vasocon Regular
naproxen T: nonnarcotic analgesic, antipyretic, anti-inflammatory P: nonsteroidal anti-inflammatory	Apo-Naproxen†, Naprosyn, Naxen†‡, Novonaprox†
naproxen sodium T: nonnarcotic analgesic, antipyretic, anti-inflammatory P: nonsteroidal anti-inflammatory	Anaprox, Anaprox DS, Naprogesic†
natamycin T: antifungal agent P: polyene macrolide antibiotic	Natacyn
nedocromil sodium T: antiasthmatic agent P: cromolyn derivative	Tilade
neomycin sulfate T: antibiotic P: aminoglycoside	Aural Acute*, Bacimycin Ointment*, Bacitracin-Neomycin Ointment*, Baximan Ointment*, Biotic Ophthalmic with HC Ointment*, BPN Ointment*, Colymycin-S Otic*, Cortisporin Cream*, Cortisporin Ointment*, Cortisporin Ophthalmic Ointment*, Cortisporin Ophthalmic Suspension*, Cortisporin Otic Solution Sterile*, Cortisporin Otic Suspension*, Coracin*, Cordran-N*, Cor-Oticin*, Dexacidin Products*,

---

GENERIC NAME AND CLASSIFICATIONS	TRADE NAMES
neomycin sulfate (continued)	Drotic Sterile Otic Suspension*, Epimycin A*, Maxitrol Ophthalmic*, Mitymycin*, Mycifradin†, Myciguent, Mycitracin*, Mycolog*, Necort*, Neocort*, Neocortef*, Neo-Decadron*, Neo-Decaspray*, Neo-Deltef*, Neo-Hydeltrasol*, Neomedrol*, Neo-Mixin*, Neomycin Sulfate and Bacitracin Ointment*, Neomycin Sulfate and Dexamethasone Sodium Phosphate Cream*, Neomycin Sulfate and Dexamethasone Sodium Phosphate Ophthalmic Solution*, Neomycin Sulfate and Fluocinolone Acetonide Cream*, Neomycin Sulfate and Methylprednisolone Acetate Cream*, Neomycin Sulfate and Prednisolone Ointment*, Neomycin Sulfate and Prednisolone Acetate Ophthalmic Ointment*, Neomycin Sulfate and Prednisolone Acetate Ophthalmic Suspension*, Neomycin Sulfate and Prednisolone Sodium Phosphate Ophthalmic Ointment*, Neomycin and Sulfacetamide Sodium, and Prednisolone Acetate Ophthalmic Ointment*, Neopolycin-HC*, Neosporin Ointment*, Neosulf‡, Neosynlar*, Neo-Tal*, Neothryex*, Otoreid-HC*, P.B.N. Ointment*, Tigo Ointment*, Tri-Biotic Ointment*, Trimixin*, Triple Antibiotic Ointment*
neostigmine bromide T: muscle stimulant P: cholinesterase inhibitor	Prostigmin Bromide
neostigmine methylsulfate T: muscle stimulant P: cholinesterase inhibitor	Prostigmin
netilmicin sulfate T: antibiotic P: aminoglycoside	Netromycin
nicardipine T: antianginal, antihypertensive P: calcium channel blocker	Cardene

GENERIC NAME AND CLASSIFICATIONS	TRADE NAMES
niclosamide T: anthelmintic P: salicylanilide	Niclocide, Yomesan‡
nicotine polacrilex (nicotine resin complex) T: smoking cessation aid P: nicotinic agonist	Nicorette
nifedipine T: antianginal P: calcium channel blocker	Adalat, Adalat P.A.†, Apo-Nifed, Novo-Nifedin, Procardia, Procardia XL
nimodipine T: cerebral vasodilator P: calcium channel blocker	Nimotop
nitrofurantoin macrocrystals T: urinary tract antiseptic P: nitrofuran	Macrodantin
nitrofurantoin microcrystals T: urinary tract antiseptic P: nitrofuran	Apo-Nitrofurantoin†, Furadantin, Furalan, Furan, Furanite, Macrodantin, Nephronex†, Nitrofan, Novofuran†
nitrofurazone T: topical antibacterial P: synthetic antibacterial nitrofuran derivative	Eldezol*, Furacin, Furacin-E Urethral Inserts*
nitroglycerin (glyceryl trinitrate) T: antianginal, vasodilator P: nitrate	Deponit, Klavikordal, Niong, Nitradisc‡, Nitro-Bid, Nitro-Bid I.V., Nitrocap, Nitrocap T.D., Nitrocine, Nitrodisc, Nitro-Dur, Nitro-Dur II, Nitrodyl-B*, Nitrogard, Nitrogard SR, Nitrol, Nitrolate Ointment‡, Nitrolin, Nitrolingual, Nitrol TSAR, Nitronet, Nitrong, Nitrong S.R., Nitrospan, Nitrostat, Nitrostat I.V., Nitrotym-Plus*, Nitrovas*, NTS, Nyomin*, Peritrate with Nitroglycerin*, Transderm-Nitro, Tridil
nitroprusside sodium T: antihypertensive P: vasodilator	Nipride, Nitropress
nizatidine T: antiulcer agent P: histamine H_2-receptor antagonist	Axid

T Therapeutic classification.   P Pharmacologic classification.

GENERIC NAME AND CLASSIFICATIONS	TRADE NAMES
norepinephrine bitartrate (levarterenol bitartrate) T: vasopressor P: direct-acting adrenergic	Levophed
norethindrone T: contraceptive P: progestin	Brevicon 21 & 28*, Micronor, Modicon 21 & 28*, Norinyl*, Norinyl-L Fe 28*, Norlutin, Nor-Q.D., Ortho Novum 21 & 28*, Ortho Novum 7/7/7-21 & 28*, Ortho Novum 10/11-21 & 28*, Ortho Novum 1/50*, Ortho Novum 1/80*, Ovcon-35 & 50*
norethindrone acetate T: contraceptive P: progestin	Aygestin, Aygestin Cycle Pack, Loestrin 1/20*, Loestrin 1.5/30*, Norlestrin*, Norlestrin Fe Tab*, Norlutate
norfloxacin T: broad-spectrum antibiotic P: fluoroquinolone	Noroxin
norgestrel T: contraceptive P: progestin	Lo/Ovral*, Ovral*, Ovrette
nortriptyline hydrochloride T: antidepressant P: tricyclic antidepressant	Aventyl, Pamelor
novobiocin sodium T: antibiotic P: polycyclic antibiotic	Albamycin
nylidrin hydrochloride T: peripheral vasodilator P: beta-adrenergic agonist	Adrin, Arlidin, Arlidin Forte†, PMS Nylidrin†
nystatin T: antifungal P: polyene macrolide	Achrostatin-V*, Co-Mycin*, Declostatin*, Mycolog*, Mycostatin, Nadostine†, Nilstat, Nystaform*, Nystex, Tetrex-F*

---

† Available in Canada only.   ‡ Available in Australia only.   * Combination product.

GENERIC NAME AND CLASSIFICATIONS	TRADE NAMES
octreotide acetate T: somatotropic hormone P: synthetic octapeptide	Sandostatin
ofloxacin T: antibiotic P: fluoroquinolone	Floxin
olsalazine sodium T: anti-inflammatory P: salicylate	Dipentum
omeprazole T: gastric acid suppressant P: substituted benzimidazole	Prilosec
ondansetron hydrochloride T: antiemetic P: serotonin receptor antagonist	Zofran
opium tincture T: antidiarrheal P: opiate	Dia-Quel*, Opecto*, Parelixir*
opium tincture, camphorated (paregoric) T: antidiarrheal P: opiate	Duosorb*, Kaoparin*, Kapectin*, Ka-Pek with Paregoric*, Parepectolin*
orphenadrine citrate T: skeletal muscle relaxant P: diphenhydramine analog	Banflex, Flexoject, Flexon, K-Flex, Marflex, Myolin, Neocyten, Nobegesic*, Noradex, Norflex, Norgesic Forte*, O-Flex, Orflagen, Orphenate
oxacillin sodium T: antibiotic P: penicillinase-resistant penicillin	Bactocill, Prostaphlin
oxamniquine T: anthelmintic P: tetrahydroquinoline	Vansil
oxandrolone T: anabolic, anti-osteoporotic P: anabolic steroid	Anavar, Lonavar‡

T Therapeutic classification.   P Pharmacologic classification.

GENERIC NAME AND CLASSIFICATIONS	TRADE NAMES
oxazepam T: antianxiety agent, sedative-hypnotic P: benzodiazepine	Apo-Oxazepam†, Novoxapam†, Ox-Pam†, Serax, Zapex†
oxiconazole nitrate T: antifungal P: ergosterol synthesis inhibitor	Oxistat
oxidized cellulose T: local hemostatic P: polyanhydroglucuronic acid	Oxycel, Surgicel
oxtriphylline (choline theophyllinate) T: bronchodilator P: xanthine derivative	Brondecon*, Choledyl
oxybutynin chloride T: antispasmodic P: synthetic tertiary amine	Ditropan
oxycodone hydrochloride T: analgesic P: opioid	Endone‡, Percocet-5*, Roxicodone, Supeudol†, Tylox*
oxymetazoline hydrochloride T: decongestant, vasoconstrictor P: sympathomimetic agent	Afrin, Afrin Children's Strength Nose Drops, Allerest 12-Hour Nasal, Chlorphed-LA, Coricidin Nasal Mist, Dristan Long Lasting, Drixine Nasal‡, Duramist Plus, Duration, 4-Way Long-Acting Nasal, Genasal Spray, Neo-Synephrine 12 Hour, Nostrilla, NTZ Long Acting Nasal, Sinarest 12-Hour, Sinex Long-Acting, Twice-A-Day Nasal
oxymetholone T: antianemic P: anabolic steroid	Anadrol-50, Anapolon†, Anapolon 50†‡
oxymorphone hydrochloride T: analgesic P: opioid	Numorphan
oxyphenbutazone T: nonnarcotic analgesic, antipyretic, anti-inflammatory, uricosuric P: nonsteroidal anti-inflammatory	

GENERIC NAME AND CLASSIFICATIONS	TRADE NAMES
oxyphencyclimine hydro-chloride T: gastrointestinal anti-spasmodic P: anticholinergic	Daricon, Daricon-PB*, Enarax*
oxytetracycline hydro-chloride T: antibiotic P: tetracycline	E.P. Mycin, Terramycin*, Urobiotic*
oxytocin, synthetic injection T: oxytocic, lactation stimu-lant P: exogenous hormone	Oxytocin, Pitocin, Syntocinon
oxytocin, synthetic nasal solution T: oxytocic, lactation stimu-lant P: exogenous hormone	Syntocinon

P

GENERIC NAME AND CLASSIFICATIONS

TRADE NAMES

pamidronate
T: antipsoriatic agent
P: retinoid

Aredia

pancreatin
T: digestant
P: pancreatic enzyme

Dizymes Tablets, Donnazyme*, Entozyme*, Hi-Vegi-Lip Tablets, Pancreatin Enseals, Pancreatin Tablets, Pepsatal*, Phazyme*, Phazyme 95*, Phazyme-PB*

pancrelipase
T: digestant
P: pancreatic enzyme

Accelerase*, Cotazym Capsules, Cotazym-S Capsules, Creon Capsules, Festal II Tablets, Ilozyme Tablets, Ku-Zyme HP Capsules, Pancrease Capsules, Pancrease MT4, Pancrease MT10, Pancrease MT16, Viokase Powder, Viokase Tablets

pancuronium bromide
T: skeletal muscle relaxant
P: nondepolarizing
neuromuscular blocking
agent

Pavulon

papaverine hydrochloride
T: peripheral vasodilator
P: benzylisoquinoline
derivative, opiate alkaloid

Cerespan, Copavin*, Copavin Compound*, Genabid, Golacol*, Pavabid, Pavabid HP Capsulets, Pavabid Plateau Caps, Pavadel-PB*, Pavarine Spancaps, Pavasule, Pavatine, Pavatym, Paverolan Lanacaps

paramethadione
T: anticonvulsant
P: oxazolidinedione
derivative

Paradione

paramethasone acetate
T: anti-inflammatory, immunosuppressant
P: glucocorticoid

Haldrone

paromomycin sulfate
T: antibacterial, amebicide
P: aminoglycoside

Humatin

GENERIC NAME AND CLASSIFICATIONS	TRADE NAMES
pemoline T: analeptic P: oxazolidinedione derivative, central nervous system stimulant	Cylert, Cylert Chewable
penbutolol sulfate T: antihypertensive P: beta-adrenergic blocking agent	Levatol
D-penicillamine T: heavy metal antagonist, antirheumatic agent P: chelating agent	Cuprimine, Depen, D-Penamine‡
penicillin G benzathine (benzylpenicillin benzathine) T: antibiotic P: natural penicillin	Bicillin C-R*, Bicillin C-R 900/300*, Bicillin L-A, Megacillin
penicillin G potassium (benzylpenicillin potassium) T: antibiotic P: natural penicillin	Lanacillin, Megacillin†, NovoPen-G†, Pentids*, Pentids 400*, Pentids 800*, P-50†, Pfizerpen
penicillin G procaine (benzylpenicillin procaine) T: antibiotic P: natural penicillin	Ayercillin†, Bicillin C-R*, Bicillin C-R 900/300*, Crysticillin A.S., Duracillin A.S., Pfizerpen-AS, Wycillin
penicillin G sodium (benzylpenicillin sodium) T: antibiotic P: natural penicillin	Crystapen†
penicillin V (phenoxymethyl penicillin) T: antibiotic P: natural penicillin	
penicillin V potassium (phenoxymethylpenicillin potassium) T: antibiotic P: natural penicillin	Abbocillin VK‡, Apo-Pen-VK†, Beepen-VK, Betapen-VK, Cilicane VK‡, Ledercillin VK, Nadopen-V†, NovoPen-VK†, Penapar VK, Pen Vee K, PVF K†, PVK‡, Robicillin VK, V-Cillin K, VC-K, Veetids
pentaerythritol tetranitrate T: antianginal, vasodilator P: nitrate	Angijen S.C. Salmon*, Angijen #1 Salmon*, Arcotrate*, Bitrate*, Dilar, Dimycor*, Duotrate, Miltrate*, Naptrate, Penta-Cap Plus*, Penta-Tal #3*, Penta-Tal #4*, Pentritol, Pentylan,

---

T Therapeutic classification.   P Pharmacologic classification.

GENERIC NAME AND CLASSIFICATIONS	TRADE NAMES
pentaerythritol tetranitrate *(continued)*	Peritrate, Peritrate Forte†, Peritrate SA, Peritrate with Nitroglycerin*, PETN, Robam-Petn*
pentamidine isethionate T: antiprotozoal P: diamidine derivative	NebuPent, Pentam 300
pentazocine hydrochloride T: analgesic, adjunct to anesthesia P: narcotic agonist-antagonist, opioid partial agonist	Fortral‡, Talwin†
pentazocine hydrochloride and nalaxone hydrochloride T: analgesic, adjunct to anesthesia P: narcotic agonist-antagoist, opioid partial agonist	Talwin Nx
pentazocine lactate T: analgesic, adjunct to anesthesia P: narcotic agonist-antagonist, opioid partial agonist	Fortral‡, Talwin
pentobarbital T: anticonvulsant, sedative-hypnotic P: barbiturate	Cafergot-P.B.*, Nembutal, Quad-Set*
pentobarbital sodium T: anticonvulsant, sedative-hypnotic P: barbiturate	A-N-R Rectorette*, Cafergot-P.B.*, Eldonal*, Ephedrine and Nembutal 25*, Fetamin*, Homachol*, Nembutal Sodium, Novopentobarb†, Spasmasorb*
pentostatin T: antileukemic P: adenosine deaminase inhibitor	Nipent
pentoxifylline T: hemorrheologic agent P: xanthine derivative	Trental
pergolide mesylate T: antiparkinsonian agent P: dopaminergic antagonist	Permax
permethrin T: pediculocide P: synthetic pyrethroid	Nix

† Available in Canada only.   ‡ Available in Australia only.   * Combination product.

GENERIC NAME AND CLASSIFICATIONS	TRADE NAMES
perphenazine T: antipsychotic, antiemetic P: phenothiazine (piperazine derivative)	Apo-Perphenazine†, Phenazine†, Trilafon
phenacemide T: anticonvulsant P: substituted acetylurea derivative, open-chain hydantoin	Phenurone
phenazopyridine hydrochloride T: urinary analgesic P: azo dye	Azo-Cyst*, Azo-Gantanol*, Azo-Gantrisin*, Azo-Standard, Azo-Sulfisoxazole*, Baridium, Di-Azo, Eridium, Geridium, Phenazo†, Phenazodine, Pyrazodine, Pyridiate, Pyridin, Pyridium, Pyridium Plus*, Pyronium, Rosoxol-Azo*, Triursil*, Uridium*, Urisan-P*, Urobiotic*, Urodine, Urogesic*, Urotrol*, Viridium
phendimetrazine tartrate T: short-term anorexigenic agent for exogenous obesity, indirect-acting sympathomimetic amine P: amphetamine congener	Adipost, Adphen, Anorex, Bacarate, Bontril PDM, Bontril Slow Release, Dyrexan OD, Melfiat, Metra, Obalan, Obeval, Phenazine-35, Phenzine, Plegine, Prelu-2, Slyn-LL, Sprx-105, Statobex, Trimtabs, Trimstat, Wehless, Weightrol, X-Trozine, X-Trozine LA
phenelzine sulfate T: antidepressant P: monoamine oxidase inhibitor	Nardil
pheniramine maleate T: antihistamine P: propylamine-derivative antihistamine	Chexit*, Decobel*, Derma-Pax*, Inhiston, Tussagesic*, Tussaminic*, Symptrol Syrup*
phenmetrazine hydrochloride T: short-term anorexigenic agent, indirect-acting sympathomimetic amine P: amphetamine congener	Preludin
phenobarbital (phenobarbitone) T: anticonvulsant, sedative-hypnotic P: barbiturate	Alkets*, Amodrine*, Anjigen S.C. Salmon*, Anjigen #1*, Antrocol*, Apcogesic*, Arcotate #3*, Asmadrin*, Asminorel*, Aspirbar*, Banthine with Phenobarbital*, Barbelod*, Barbita,

GENERIC NAME AND CLASSIFICATIONS	TRADE NAMES
phenobarbital *(continued)*	Bellergal*, Bentyl with Phenobarbital*, Bitrate*, B.M.E.*, Brobella-P.B.*, Bronkolixr*, Bronkotab*, Cafergot P-B*, Cantril with Phenobarbital*, Cardilate-P*, Daricon-PB*, Detal*, Dilantin with Phenobarbital Kapseals*, Doloral*, Donnacin*, Donnatal*, Donnatal #2*, Donnazyme*, Eponal*, Fenatron*, Gardenal†, Glynaphen*, Haponal*, Hyonal C.T.*, Hytrona*, Isophed*, Kinesed*, Lardet*, Luminal†, Mass Donna*, Mudrane*, Mudrane GG-2*, Neogen*, Nidar*, Nilspasm*, Palbar #2*, Pamine PB*, Pavadel-PB*, Peece Kaps*, Phazyme-PB*, Probital*, Quadrinal*, Quadset*, Raudilan*, Robantaline with Phenobarbital*, RoTrim*, S.B.P.*, Scopine*, Sedamine*, Sedapar*, Sedragesic*, Setamine*, Solfoton, Sorbitate with Phenobarbital*, Spabelin*, Spasaid*, Spasmolin*, Spasquid*, Stannitol*, Synophedral*, Synophylate with Phenobarbital*, Synt-PB*, Tedral Elixir*, Tedral SA*, Theolaphen*, Ultabs*
phenobarbital sodium (phenobarbitone sodium) T: anticonvulsant, sedative-hypnotic P: barbiturate	Iso-Asminyl*, Luminal Sodium†, Nidar*, Plexonal*
phenolphthalein, white T: stimulant laxative P: anthraquinone derivative	Alophen Pills, Medilax, Modane, Modane Mild, Phenolax Wafers, Prulet
phenolphthalein, yellow T: stimulant laxative P: anthraquinone derivative	Correctol*, Disolan*, Evac-U-Gen, Evac-U-Lax, Ex-Lax*, Feen-A-Mint Gum, Feen-A-Mint Pills*, Lax-Pills
phenoxybenzamine hydrochloride T: antihypertensive for pheochromocytoma, cutaneous vasodilator P: alpha-adrenergic blocking agent	Dibenyline‡, Dibenzyline
phensuximide T: anticonvulsant P: succinimide derivative	Milontin

---

† Available in Canada only.   ‡ Available in Australia only.   * Combination product.

GENERIC NAME AND CLASSIFICATIONS	TRADE NAMES
phentermine hydrochloride T: short-term adjunctive anorexigenic agent, indirect-acting sympathomimetic amine P: amphetamine congener	Adipex-P, Dapex, Duromine‡, Fastin, Ionamin, Obe-Nix, Obephen, Obermine, Obestin, Oby-Trim, Parmine, Phentrol, Span R/D, Teramine, Unifast
phentolamine mesylate T: antihypertensive agent for pheochromocytoma, cutaneous vasodilator P: alpha-adrenergic blocking agent	Regitine, Rogitine†
phenylbutazone T: nonnarcotic analgesic, antipyretic, anti-inflammatory, uricosuric P: nonsteroidal anti-inflammatory	Apo-Phenylbutazone†, Azolid, Azolid-A*, Butazolidin, Butazolidin Alicia*, Butazone, Intrabutazone†, Novobutazone†
phenylephrine hydrochloride T: vasoconstrictor P: adrenergic	Acotus*, AK-Dilate, AK-Nefrin Ophthalmic, Alconefrin 12, Alconefrin 25, Alconefrin 50, Allerest Nasal Spray*, Anodynos Forte*, Atussin DM*, Bellafedrol A-H*, Brolade*, Burtuss*, CDM Expectorant*, Centuss*, Cerose-DM*, Chew Hist*, Codimal DM*, Colrex Compound*, Conar*, Conar-A*, Congespirin*, Cophene-PL*, Cophene-S*, Cophene-X*, Cortane*, Cortapp*, Cyclomydril Solution*, Dallergy*, Dimetane Decongestant*, Doktors, Donatussin Syrup*, Dristan 12 Hour*, Drucon*, Duration, Efricel 1/8%*, Efricon Expectorant*, Emagin Forte*, Entex*, Extendryl*, Fendol*, 4-Way Nasal Spray*, Guistrey*, Histaspan-D*, Histaspan-Plus*, Histavadrin*, Hycoff-A*, I-Phrine 2.5%, Isopto Frin, Kiddies Sialco*, Koryza*, Marhist*, Mydfrin*, Nasahist*, N-D Gesic*, Neo-Synephrine, Niltuss*, Nostril, Novahistine Expectorant*, Pediacof*, Phenahist-TR*, Phenatuss*, Phenergran-D*, Phenylzin*, P.M.P*, Polyectin*, Prednefrin-S*, Prefin A*, Prefin Z*, Prefrin Liquifilm, Proclan VC Expectorant*, Proclan VC Expectorant with Codeine*, Pyma*, Pyristan*,

---

T Therapeutic classification.   P Pharmacologic classification.

GENERIC NAME AND CLASSIFICATIONS	TRADE NAMES
phenylephrine hydrochloride *(continued)*	Quelidrine*, Rentuss*, Rhinall, Rhinall-10, Rhinogesic*, Rinocidin*, Salphenyl*, Scotnord*, Scotuf*, Scotuss*, Shertuss Liquid*, Sialco*, Sinarex Aerosol*, Sinex*, Sinovan Timed*, Sinucol*, Spantuss*, Spec-T Sore Throat Decongestant Lozenges*, St. Joseph Measured Dose Nasal Decongestant, Symptrol Syrup*, Thor Syrup*, Tonecol*, Trihistin Expectorant*, Turbilixir*, Turbispan Leisurecaps*, Tusquelin*, Tussar-DM*, Tympagesic*, Valihist*, Vasosulf*, Vernacel*
phenylpropanolamine hydrochloride T: nasal decongestant, antiobesity agent, agent in treatment of stress incontinence and to correct retrograde ejaculation in patients with diabetic neuropathy P: synthetic phenylisopropanolamine sympathomimetic	Allerest*, Alumadrine*, Anti Tussive*, Atussin-DM*, A.R.M.*, Bayer Children's Cold Tablets*, Bayer Cough Syrup for Children*, BC Powder*, Bobid*, Bowman Cold*, BQ Cold*, Breacol Cough Medicine*, Bro-Tane Expectorant*, Bur-Tuss*, Capahist-DMH*, Chlordri*, Conex*, Congespirin*, Contac 12 Hour*, Cophene-PL*, Cophene-S*, Cophene-X*, Coricidin Sinus Headache*, Cortane*, Cortapp*, Decobel*, Decojen*, Dehist*, Demazin*, Dezest*, Dimetane Expectorant-DC*, Dimetane Extendtabs*, Drinophen*, Entex*, Fitacol*, 4-Way Nasal Spray*, 4-Way Tabs*, Hall's Mentho-Lyptus Decongestant Cough Formula*, Hista-Vadrin*, Histogesic*, Histosal #2*, Infantuss*, Kleer*, Koryza*, Lanatuss Expectorant*, Nasahist*, Nilcol*, Nolamine*, Ornex*, Partuss-A*, Phenahist Injection*, Phenahist-TR*, Polyectin*, Pyristan*, Rentuss*, Rhinex*, Robitussin-CF*, Rohist-D*, Rolanade*, Rymed*, Saleto-D*, Santussin*, Scotuss*, Sinarest*, Sine-Off*, Sinubid*, Sinucin*, Spec-T Sore Throat Decongestant*, St. Joseph Cold Tabs*, Symptrol*, Triaminic Allergy Tabs*, Triaminic Chewables*, Triaminic Cold*, Triaminic DM Cough Formula*, Triaminic Expectorant*, Triaminic Expectorant with Codeine*, Triaminicin*, Triaminic Multi-Symp-
(continued)

GENERIC NAME AND CLASSIFICATIONS	TRADE NAMES
phenylpropanolamine hydrochloride *(continued)*	tom*, Tri-Histin Expectorant*, Trind-DM*, Turbilixir*, Turbispan Leisurecaps*, Tusquelin*, Tussaminic*, Tussagesic*
phenytoin T: anticonvulsant P: hydantoin derivative	Dilantin, Dilantin Infatabs, Dilantin-30 Pediatric, Dilantin-125
phenytoin sodium T: anticonvulsant P: hydantoin derivative	Dilantin, Dilantin with Phenobarbital*
phenytoin sodium (extended) T: anticonvulsant P: hydantoin derivative	Dilantin Kapseals
phenytoin sodium (prompt) T: anticonvulsant P: hydantoin derivative	Di-Phen, Diphenylan
physostigmine T: antimuscarinic, antidote, antiglaucoma agent P: cholinesterase inhibitor	Eserine, Isopto-Eserine
physostigmine salicylate (eserine) T: antimuscarinic antidote, antiglaucoma agent P: cholinesterase inhibitor	Antilirium, Atrophysine*, Isopto P-Es*, Phyatromine-H*
pilocarpine hydrochloride T: miotic P: cholinergic agonist	Adsorbocarpine, E-Carpine*, E-Pilo*, Isopto Carpine, Isopto-PEs*, Miocarpine†, Ocusert Pilo, Pilocar, Pilocel, Pilomiotin, Pilopine HS, Pilopt‡
pilocarpine nitrate T: miotic P: cholinergic agonist	Pilofrin Liquifilm*, P.V. Carpine Liquifilm
pimozide T: antipsychotic P: diphenylbutylpiperidine	Orap
pinacidil T: antihypertensive P: vasodilator	Pindac
pindolol T: antihypertensive P: beta-adrenergic blocking agent	Barbloc‡, Visken

T Therapeutic classification.   P Pharmacologic classification.

GENERIC NAME AND CLASSIFICATIONS	TRADE NAMES
pipecuronium bromide T: skeletal muscle relaxant P: nondepolarizing neuromuscular blocking agent	Arduan
piperacillin sodium T: antibiotic P: extended-spectrum penicillin, acyclamino-penicillin	Pipracil, Pipril‡
piperazine adipate T: anthelmintic P: piperazine	Entacyl†
piperazine citrate T: anthelmintic P: piperazine	Antepar, Bryrel, Pin-Tega Tabs, Pipril, Ta-Verm, Veriga†, Vermirex†, Vermizine
pirbuterol T: bronochodilator P: beta-adrenergic agonist	Maxair
piroxicam T: nonnarcotic analgesic, antipyretic, anti-inflammatory P: nonsteroidal anti-inflammatory	Apo-Piroxicam†, Feldene, Novopirocam†
plague vaccine T: bacterial vaccine P: vaccine	
plasma protein fraction T: plasma volume expander P: blood derivative	Plasmanate, Plasma-Plex, Plasmatein, Protenate
plicamycin (mithramycin) T: antineoplastic, hypocalcemic agent P: antibiotic antineoplastic (cell cycle–phase nonspecific)	Mithracin
pneumococcal vaccine, polyvalent T: bacterial vaccine P: vaccine	Pneumovax 23, Pnu-Imune 23
podofilox T: keratolytic P: antimitotic	Condylox

† Available in Canada only.   ‡ Available in Australia only.   * Combination product.

GENERIC NAME AND CLASSIFICATIONS	TRADE NAMES
poliovirus vaccine, live, oral, trivalent T: viral vaccine P: vaccine	Orimune Trivalent
polyethylene glycol-electrolyte solution T: bowel evacuant P: electrolyte solution	Colovage, CoLyte, Glycoprep‡, GoLYTELY, OCL Solution
polymyxin B sulfate T: antibiotic P: polymyxin antibiotic	Aerosporin, Aural Acute*, Baximan Ointment*, Biotic with Hydrocortisone Ointment*, BPN Ointment*, Chloromyxin B*, Coracin Ointment*, Cortisporin Cream*, Cortisporin Ointment*, Cortisporin Ophthalmic Ointment*, Cortisporin Ophthalmic Suspension*, Cortisporin Otic Solution Sterile*, Cortisporin Otic Suspension*, Dexacidin*, Drotic Sterile Otic Solution*, Epimycin A*, Maxitrol*, Mity Mycin Ointment*, Mycitracin*, Neomixin*, Neopolycin-HC Ointment*, Neosporin Ointment*, Neotal*, Neo-Thrycex*, Opthocort*, Otobiotic*, Otoreid-HC*, P.B.N. Ointment*, Polysporin*, Pyocidin-Otic*, Statrol*, Statrol Sterile Ophthalmic Ointment*, Terramycin*, Tigo Ointment*, Tri-Biotic Ointment*, Tri-Bow Ointment*, Triple Antibiotic Ointment*
polythiazide T: diuretic, antihypertensive P: thiazide diuretic	Minizide*, Renese, Renese-R*
potassium acetate T: therapeutic agent for electrolyte balance P: potassium supplement	
potassium bicarbonate T: therapeutic agent for electrolyte balance P: potassium supplement	K+Care ET, Klor-Con/EF, K-Lyte, Quic-K
potassium chloride T: therapeutic agent for electrolyte balance P: potassium supplement	Dacriose*, K+Care, K+10, Kaochlor 10%, Kaochlor S-F 10%, Kaon-Cl, Kaon-Cl 20%, Kato Powder, Kay Ciel, K-Lease, K-Lor, Klor-10%, Klor-Con, Klorvess, Klotrix, K-Lyte/Cl, K-Tab, Micro-K Extencaps, M-Z

T Therapeutic classification.   P Pharmacologic classification.

GENERIC NAME AND CLASSIFICATIONS	TRADE NAMES
potassium chloride (*continued*)	Drops*, Naturetin W-K Tabs*, Rautrax-N Modified*, SK-Potassium Chloride, Slow-K, Swim-Eye Drops*, Ten-K
potassium gluconate T: therapeutic agent for electrolyte balance P: potassium supplement	Kaon Liquid, Kaon Tablets, Kayliker, K-G Elixir, Kolyum*, Potassium Rougier†
potassium guaiacolsulfonate T: expectorant P: electrolyte	Antitussive*, Conex, Efricon Expectorant*, Formadrin*, Partuss*, Pinex Regular, Proclan Expectorant with Codeine*, Proclan VC Expectorant with Codeine*
potassium iodide T: antihyperthyroid agent, expectorant P: electrolyte	Bricolide*, Colsalide*, Elixophyllin KI*, Iodo-Niacin*, Isophed*, KIE*, Mudrane*, Mudrane-2*, Pediacof*, Pima, Quadrinal*, TSG Croup Liquid*, TSG-KI Elixir*
potassium iodide, saturated solution (SSKI), strong iodine solution (Lugol's solution) T: expectorant, antihyperthyroid agent P: iodine solution	
pralidoxime chloride (pyridine-2-aldoxime methochloride; 2-PAM) T: antidote P: quaternary ammonium oxime	Protopam Chloride
pramoxine hydrochloride T: topical local anesthetic P: unclassified local anesthetic	Dermarex*, Epifoam*, Hydrocort*, 1+1-F Creme*, Otocalm-H Ear Drops*, Otostan HC*, Prax, Proctofoam, Proctofoam HC*, Sherform-HC*, Steraform-HC*, Tronothane Hydrochloride, V-Cort*
pravastatin sodium T: antilipemic P: HMG CoA reductase inhibitor	Pravachol
prazepam T: antianxiety agent P: benzodiazepine	Centrax

GENERIC NAME AND CLASSIFICATIONS	TRADE NAMES
praziquantel T: anthelmintic P: pyrazinoisoquinoline	Biltricide
prazosin hydrochloride T: antihypertensive P: alpha-adrenergic blocking agent	Minipress
prednisolone T: anti-inflammatory, immunosuppressant P: synthetic glucocorticoid	Cetapred Ophthalmic Ointment*, Chloroptic-P*, Cortalone, Delta-Cortef, Deltasolone‡, Fernisolone-B*, Isopto Cetapred*, Neo-Deltef*, Novo-prednisolone†, Panafcortelone†, Predoxide*, Prelone, Sarcogesic*, Solone‡
prednisolone acetate T: anti-inflammatory, immunosuppressant P: synthetic glucocorticoid	Articulose, Blephamide Liquifilm*, Blephamide S.O.P.*, Cetapred Ophthalmic Ointment*, Key-Pred, Metimyd*, Neomycin Sulfate and Prednisolone Acetate Ointment*, Neomycin Sulfate and Prednisolone Acetate Ophthalmic Ointment*, Neomycin Sulfate and Prednisolone Acetate Ophthalmic Suspension*, Neomycin Sulfate and Prednisolone Acetate, and Sulfacetamide Sodium Ophthalmic Ointment*, Niscort, Panacort R-P*, Predaject, Predalone, Predate, Predcor, Predicort, Predoxide*, Solu-Pred*, Vasocidin*
prednisolone acetate (suspension) T: anti-inflammatory, immunosuppressant P: synthetic glucocorticoid	Econopred Ophthalmic, Econopred Plus Ophthalmic, Pred-Forte, Pred Mild Ophthalmic
prednisolone sodium phosphate T: anti-inflammatory, immunosuppressant P: synthetic glucocorticoid	Codesol, Hydeltrasol, Key-Pred-SP, Neo-Hydeltrasol*, Neomycin Sulfate and Prednisolone Sodium Phosphate Ointment*, Optimyd*, Panacort R-P8, Pediapred, Predate-S, Predicort RP, Predsol Retention Enema‡, Predsol Suppositories‡, P.S.P. IV Injection*, Solu-Pred*, Vasocidin*
prednisolone sodium phosphate (solution) T: anti-inflammatory, immunosuppressant P: synthetic glucocorticoid	AK-Pred, Hydeltrasol Ophthalmic, Inflamase Forte, Inflamase Ophthalmic, Ocu-Pred, Predsol Eye Drops‡

GENERIC NAME AND CLASSIFICATIONS	TRADE NAMES
prednisolone steaglate T: anti-inlammatory, immunosuppressant P: synethetic glucocorticoid	Sintisone‡
prednisolone tebutate T: anti-inflammatory, immunosuppressant P: glucocorticoid, mineralocorticoid	Hydeltra-TBA, Metalone-TBA, Nor-Pred TBA, Predalone TBA, Predate TBA, Predcor TBA, Prednisol TBA
prednisone T: anti-inflammatory, immunosuppressant P: adrenocorticoid	Apo-Prednisone†, Deltasone, Histone*, Liquid Pred, Meticorten, Novo-prednisone†, Orasone, Panafcort‡, Panasol, Prednicen-M, Prednisone Intensol, Prednefrin-S*, Sone‡, Sterapred, Winpred†
primaquine phosphate T: antimalarial P: 8-aminoquinoline	
primidone T: anticonvulsant P: barbiturate analog	Apo-Primidone†, Myidone, Mysoline, Sertan†
probenecid T: uricosuric agent P: sulfonamide derivative	Amcill-GC*, Benemid, Benn, Benn-C Tab*, Benuryl†, Colbenemid*, Poly-cillin-PRB*, Principen with Probenecid*, Probalan, Probampacin*, Robenecid, Robenecid with Colchicine*
probucol T: cholesterol lowering agent P: bis-phenol derivative	Lorelco, Lurselle‡
procainamide hydrochloride T: ventricular antiarrhythmic, supraventricular antiarrhythmic P: procaine derivative	Procan SR, Promine, Pronestyl, Pronestyl-SR, Rhythmin
procaine hydrochloride T: local anesthetic P: procaine derivative	Glukor*, Horm-Triad*, Novocain
procarbazine hydrochloride T: antineoplastic P: antibiotic antineoplastic (cell cycle–phase specific, S phase)	Matulane, Natulan‡

GENERIC NAME AND CLASSIFICATIONS	TRADE NAMES
prochlorperazine T: antipsychotic, antiemetic, antianxiety agent P: phenothiazine (piperazine derivative)	Compazine, Iso-Perazine*, Stemetil‡
prochlorperazine edisylate T: antipsychotic, antiemetic, antianxiety agent P: phenothiazine (piperazine derivative)	Compazine
prochlorperazine maleate T: antipsychotic, antianxiety agent P: phenothiazine (piperazine derivative)	Anti-Naus‡, Chlorpazine, Compazine, Isoperazine*, Stemetil‡
procyclidine hydrochloride T: antiparkinsonian agent P: anticholinergic	Kemadrin, PMS Procyclidine†, Pro-cyclid†
progesterone T: progestin, contraceptive P: progestin	Duovin-S*, Gesterol 50, Horm-Triad*, Pro-Estrone*, Proestrone*, Pro-gestaject, Progestilin†, Progex*, Tripole-F*
promazine hydrochloride T: antipsychotic, antiemetic P: aliphatic phenothiazine	Sparine
promethazine hydrochloride T: antiemetic and antivertigo agent, antihistamine (H_1-receptor antagonist), sedative and adjunct to analgesics P: phenothiazine derivative	Anergan 25, Anergan 50, Histanil†, K-Phen, Mallergan, Mepergan*, Pentazine, Phenameth, Phenazine 25, Phenazine 50, Phencen-50, Phenergan, Phenergan-D*, Phenergan-Fortis, Phenergan-Plain, Phenergan-VC Expectorant*, Phenoject-50, PMS-Promethazine†, Proclan Expectorant with Codeine*, Proclan VC Expectorant with Codeine*, Pro-50, Prometh-25, Prometh-50, Promethegan, Prothazine‡, Prothazine-25, Prothazine-50, Prothazine Plain, Remsed, Rolamethazine VC Expectorant with Codeine*, V-Gan-25, V-Gan-50
propafenone hydrochloride T: antiarrhythmic (Class IC) P: sodium channel antagonist	Rythmol

GENERIC NAME AND CLASSIFICATIONS	TRADE NAMES
propantheline bromide T: antimuscarinic, gastrointestinal antispasmodic P: anticholinergic	Norpanth, Pantheline‡, Pro-Banthine, Pro-Banthine with Dartal*, Probital*, Propanthel†, Robantaline with Phenobarbital*
proparacaine hydrochloride T: local anesthetic P: local anesthetic	Alcaine, Ophthaine, Ophthetic
propofol T: anesthetic P: phenol derivative	Diprivan
propoxyphene hydrochloride (dextropropoxyphene hydrochloride) T: analgesic P: opioid	Darvon, Darvon Compound-65*, Darvon with Aspirin*, Dolene, Dolene AP-65*, Dolene Compound-65*, Doraphen, Doraphen Compound-65*, Doxaphene, Novopropoxyn†, Pro-Pox, Propoxycon, 642†
propoxyphene napsylate (dextropropoxyphene napsylate) T: analgesic P: opioid	Darvocet-N, Darvon-N, Doloxene‡, Doloxene Co‡
propranolol hydrochloride T: antihypertensive, antianginal, antiarrhythmic; adjunctive therapy of migraine, myocardial infarction P: beta-adrenergic blocking agent	Apo-Propranolol†, Deralin‡, Detensol†, Inderal, Inderal LA, Inderide*, Ipran, Novopranol†, PMS-Propranolol†
propylthiouracil (PTU) T: antihyperthyroid agent P: thyroid hormone antagonist	Propyl-Thyracil†
protamine sulfate T: heparin antagonist P: antidote	
protriptyline hydrochloride T: antidepressant P: tricyclic antidepressant	Triptil†, Vivactil
pseudoephedrine hydrochloride T: decongestant P: adrenergic	Actifed*, Actifed-C Syrup*, Allerest*, Alumadrine*, Ambenyl-D*, Atridine*, Brexin*, Cenafed, Children's Sudafed Liquid, Codimal*, Comtrex Cough Formula*, Congestac*, Cophene #2*, Co-Tylenol*, Decofed, *(continued)*

---

† Available in Canada only.   ‡ Available in Australia only.   * Combination product.

pseudoephedrine hydro-chloride *(continued)*

Deconamine*, Dilorbron*, Dimacol*, Dorcol Children's Decongestant, Eltor†, Excedrine*, Fedahist*, Fedrazil*, Genaphed, Guiatuss DAC*, Halofed, Isolclor*, Kronofed*, NeoFed, Novafed*, Novahistine DH*, Novahistine DMX*, Novahistine Expectorant*, Nyquil*, Ornex Cold†, Pediacare Infant's Oral Decongestant Drops, Phenergran D*, Phenergran DAC*, Phenergran PE*, Pseudofrin†, Pseudogest, Robidrine, Rondec-DM*, Rymed*, Ryna*, Ryna-C*, Sine-Aid*, Sine-Off*, Sinufed, Sinutab*, Sudafed, Sudafed Cough Syrup*, Sudafed Plus*, Sudafed 12-Hour, Sudrin, Sufedrin, Super Anahist*, Triaminic Night Lite Cold*, Tussafed Expectorant*, Vicks Daycare*, Vicks Formula 44*, Wal-Phed*

pseudoephedrine sulfate
T: decongestant
P: adrenergic

Afrinol Repetabs, Chlor-Trimeton Decongestant*, Disophrol Chrontabs*, Polarmine Expectorant*

psyllium
T: bulk laxative
P: adsorbent

Cillium, Konsyl, Metamucil, Metamucil Instant Mix, Metamucil Sugar Free, Naturacil, Perdiem*, Perdiem Plain, Siblin, Syllact

pyrantel embonate
T: anthelmintic
P: pyrimidine derivative

Anthel‡, Combantrin‡, Early Bird‡

pyrantel pamoate
T: anthelmintic
P: pyrimidine derivative

Antiminth, Combantrin†

pyrazinamide
T: antituberculosis agent
P: synthetic pyrazine analog of nicotinamide

PMS Pyrazinamide†, Tebrazid†, Zinamide‡

pyrethrins
T: pediculicide
P: pyrethrin, piperonyl butoxide and petroleum distillate combination

A-200 Pyrinate, Barc, Pyrinyl, RID, TISIT, Triple X

pyridostigmine bromide
T: muscle stimulant
P: cholinesterase inhibitor

Mestinon, Mestinon Supraspan†, Mestinon Timespan, Regonol

pyrimethamine   Daraprim, Fansidar*
T: antimalarial
P: aminopyrimidine
derivative (folic acid antagonist)

pyrimethamine with sul-   Fansidar
fadoxine
T: antimalarial agent
P: folate antagonist, sulfonamide combination

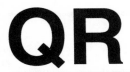

GENERIC NAME AND CLASSIFICATIONS	TRADE NAMES
quazepam T: hypnotic P: benzodiazepine	Doral
quinacrine hydrochloride (mepacrine hydrochloride) T: anthelmintic, anti-protozoal, antimalarial P: acridine derivative	Atabrine
quinapril T: antihypertensive P: angiotensin-converting en-zyme inhibitor	Accupril
quinestrol T: estrogen replacement P: estrogen	Estrovis
quinethazone T: diuretic, antihypertensive P: quinazoline derivative (thi-azide-like) diuretic	Aquamox‡, Hydromox, Hydromox-R*
quinidine bisulfate (66.4% quinidine base) T: ventricular antiarrhyth-mic, supraventricular antiar-rhythmic, atrial antitachy-arrhythmic P: cinchona alkaloid	Biquin Durules†, Kinidin Durules‡
quinidine gluconate (62% quinidine base) T: ventricular antiarrhyth-mic, supraventricular antiar-rhythmic, atrial antitachy-arrhythmic P: cinchona alkaloid	Duraquin, Quinaglute Dura-Tabs, Quinalan, Quinate†
quinidine polygalacturon-ate (60.5% quinidine base) T: ventricular antiarrhyth-mic, supraventricular antiar-rhythmic, atrial antitachy-arrhythmic P: cinchona alkaloid	Cardioquin

---

T Therapeutic classification.   P Pharmacologic classification.

GENERIC NAME AND CLASSIFICATIONS	TRADE NAMES
quinidine sulfate (83% quinidine base) T: ventricular antiarrhythmic, supraventricular antiarrhythmic, atrial antitachyarrhythmic P: cinchona alkaloid	Apo-Quinidine†, CinQuin, Novoquindin†, Quine, Quinidex Extentabs, Quinora
quinine bisulfate (quinine bisulphate) T: antimalarial, skeletal muscle relaxant P: cinchona alkaloid	Bi-Chinine‡, Biquinate‡, Myoquin‡, Quinbisul‡
quinine sulfate (quinine sulphate) T: antimalarial, skeletal muscle relaxant P: cinchona alkaloid	Chinine‡, Coryza*, Legatrin, Myodyne*, Novoquinine†, Quinamm, Quinate‡, Quindan, Quine-200, Quine-300, Quinoctal‡, Quiphile, Strema*, Sulquin‡
rabies immune globulin, human T: rabies prophylaxis agent P: immune serum	Hyperab, Imogam
rabies vaccine, human diploid cell (HDCV) T: viral vaccine P: vaccine	Imovax
radioactive iodine (sodium iodide) ^{131}I T: antihyperthyroid agent P: thyroid hormone antagonist	Iodotope Therapeutic, Sodium Iodide ^{131}I Therapeutic
ramipril T: antihypertensive P: angiotensin-converting enzyme inhibitor	Altace
ranitidine hydrochloride T: antiulcer agent P: histamine$_2$-receptor antagonist	Zantac
rauwolfia serpentina T: antihypertensive P: rauwolfia alkaloid, peripherally acting adrenergic-blocking agent	Maxitrate with Rauwolfia*, Raudilan*, Raudixin, Rautrax*, Rautrax-N*, Rauverid, Rauzide*, Wolfina

GENERIC NAME AND CLASSIFICATIONS	TRADE NAMES

rescinnamine
T: antihypertensive
P: rauwolfia alkaloid, peripherally acting adrenergic-blocking agent

Moderil

reserpine
T: antihypertensive, antipsychotic
P: rauwolfia alkaloid, peripherally acting adrenergic-blocking agent

Demi-Regroton*, Diupres*, Harbolin*, Hydromox R*, Hydropres-25 & 50*, Hydroserp*, Hydroserpine*, Hydrotensin-50*, Hyperserp*, Mallopress*, Metatensin*, Novoreserpine†, Regroton*, Renese-R*, Salutensin*, Salutensin-Demi*, Ser-Ap-Es*, Serapine*, Serpalan, Serpasil, Serpasil-Apresoline*, Serpasil-Esidrix*, Thia-Serp-25 & 50*, Thia-Serpa-Zine*, Unipres*

Rh$_o$ (D) immune globulin, human
T: anti-Rh$_o$ (D)-positive prophylaxis agent
P: immune serum

Gamulin Rh, HypRho-D, MICRhoGAM, Mini-Gamulin Rh, Rhesonativ, RhoGAM

ribavirin
T: antiviral agent
P: synthetic nucleoside

Virazole

rifampin (rifampicin)
T: antituberculosis agent
P: semisynthetic rifamycin B derivative (macrocyclic antibiotic)

Rifadin, Rimactane*, Rimycin‡, Rofact†

Ringer's injection
T: electrolyte and fluid replenishment
P: electrolyte solution

Ringer's injection, lactated (Hartmann's solution; Ringer's lactate solution)
T: electrolyte and fluid replenishment
P: electrolyte-carbohydrate solution

ritodrine hydrochloride
T: adjunctive agent in suppression of preterm labor
P: beta-receptor agonist

Yutopar

T Therapeutic classification.   P Pharmacologic classification.

GENERIC NAME AND CLASSIFICATIONS	TRADE NAMES
rubella and mumps virus vaccine, live T: viral vaccine P: vaccine	Biavax II
rubella virus vaccine, live attenuated T: viral vaccine P: vaccine	Lirubel*, Lirutrin*, Meruvax II, M-M-R Vaccine*, M-R-Vax*

S

GENERIC NAME AND CLASSIFICATIONS	TRADE NAMES
salicylamide T: nonnarcotic analgesic, antipyretic, anti-inflammatory P: nonsteroidal anti-inflammatory	Akes-N-Pain*, Anodynos Forte*, Arthralgen*, Bisalate*, Centuss*, Dengesic*, Duoprin*, Emagrin*, Emagrin Professional Strength*, F.C.A.H.*, Fendol*, Histapco*, Indogesic*, Kiddies Sialco*, Metrogesic*, Myocalm*, Panritis*, Partuss-A*, Presalin*, Pyranistan*, Renpap*, Rhinex*, Rhinogesic*, S.A.C. Sinus*, Saleto*, Saleto-D*, Salocol*, Salphenyl*, Scotgesic*, Sedacane*, Sedalgesic*, Sedragesic*, Sialco*
salsalate T: nonnarcotic analgesic, antipyretic, anti-inflammatory P: salicylate	Arthra-G, Disalcid, Mono-Gesic, Salflex, Salgesic, Salsitab
sargramostim T: immune stimulant P: biological response modifier; colony stimulating factor	Leukine
scopolamine (hyoscine) T: antimuscarinic, antiemetic-antivertigo agent, antiparkinsonian agent, cycloplegic mydriatic P: anticholinergic	Transderm-Scop, Transderm-V†, Urogesic*
scopolamine butylbromide (hyoscine butylbromide) T: antimuscarinic, antiemetic-antivertigo agent, antiparkinsonian agent, cycloplegic mydriatic P: anticholinergic	Buscospan†‡
scopolamine hydrobromide (hyoscine hydrobromide) T: antimuscarinic, antiemetic-antivertigo agent, antiparkinsonian agent, cycloplegic mydriatic P: anticholinergic	Aridol*, Azo-Cyst*, Barbeloid*, Brobella-P.B.*, Butabell HMB*, DeTal*, Donnacin*, Donnatal*, Donnatal #2*, Donnazyme*, Eldonal*, Enterex*, Fenatron*, Haponal*, Hyonal C.T.*, Hyonatol*, Hyonatol B-Elixir*, Hytrona*, Isopto Hydro-

---

T Therapeutic classification.   P Pharmacologic classification.

GENERIC NAME AND CLASSIFICATIONS	TRADE NAMES
scopolamine hydrobromide (*continued*)	bromide*, Isopto Hyosine, Kapigam*, Kinesed*, Koryza*, Mass-Donna*, Nilspasm*, Palbar #2*, Palsorb Improved*, Pedo-Sol*, Peece*, Plexonal*, Scopine*, Sedamine*, Sedapar*, Setamine*, Sidonna*, Spabelin*, Spasaid*, Spasmolin*, Spasquid*, Stannitol*
secobarbital sodium T: sedative-hypnotic, anticonvulsant P: barbiturate	Amoseco*, Monosyl*, Nidar*, Novosecobarb†, Quad-Set*, S.B.P.*, Seconal Sodium, Sedalgesic*, Tuinal*
selegiline hydrochloride (L-deprenyl hydrochloride) T: antiparkinsonian agent P: monoamine-oxidase inhibitor	Eldepryl
senna T: stimulant laxative P: anthraquinone derivative	Black-Draught, Gentalax S*, Perdiem*, Sarolax*, Senokapp-DDS*, Senokot, Senokot-S*, X-Prep Liquid
sertraline T: antidepressant P: serotonin uptake inhibitor	Zoloft
silver nitrate 1% T: ophthalmic antiseptic; topical cauterizing agent P: heavy metal (silver compound)	
silver sulfadiazine T: topical antibacterial P: synthetic anti-infective	Flamazine†, Flint SSD, Silvadene, Thermazene
simethicone T: antiflatulent P: dispersant	Di-Gel*, Extra Strength Gas-X, Gas-X, Gelusil*, Kinesed*, Laxsil*, Maalox*, Maalox Plus*, Mylanta*, Mylanta II*, Mylicon-80, Mylicon-125, Ovol-40†, Ovol-80†, Phazyme*, Phazyme 55, Phazyme 95*, Phazyme 125, Phazyme-PB*, Sidonna*, Silain, Silain-Gel*, Simeco*, Simethox*
simvastatin T: antilipemic P: HMG CoA reductase inhibitor	Zocor

---

GENERIC NAME AND CLASSIFICATIONS	TRADE NAMES
sodium benzoate and sodium phenylacetate T: urea cycle enzymopathy treatment adjunct P: enzyme substrates	Ucephan
sodium bicarbonate T: systemic and urinary alkalinizer, systemic hydrogen ion buffer, oral antacid P: alkalinizing agent	Alka-Seltzer Plus*, Anacholric A*
sodium cellulose phosphate T: antiurolithic P: ion exchange resin	Calcibind
sodium chloride T: sodium and chloride replacement P: electrolyte	Bromidrosis Crystals*, Calpholac*, Calphosan*, Cogentin*, Cor-Oticin*, Garamycin Ophthalmic Solution*, Glaucon*, Tostestro*, Vasocon-A Ophthalmic Solution*
sodium chloride, hypertonic T: treatment of corneal edema, diagnostic aid P: ophthalmic hypertonic sodium chloride agent	Adsorbonac Ophthalmic Solution, AK-NaCl, Muro-128 Ointment, Sodium Chloride Ointment 5%
sodium fluoride T: dental caries prophylactic P: trace mineral	Fluorac*, Fluor-A-Day†, Fluoritab, Flura, Flura-Drops, Karidium, Luride, Mulvidren-F*, Pediaflor, Phos-Flur, So-Flo*, Tri-Vi-Flor*
sodium fluoride, topical T: dental caries preventative, adjunctive treatment of osteoporosis P: unclassified	ACT, Checkmate, Fluorigard, Fluorinse, Flura-Drops, Gel-Kam, Gel-Tin, Gel II, Home Treatment Fluoride Gelution, Karigel, Karigel-N, Listermint with Fluoride, Minute-Gel, Point-Two, PreviDent, Stop, Thera-Flur, Thera-Flur N
sodium lactate T: systemic alkalizer P: alkalinizing agent	
sodium phosphates (sodium phosphate and sodium biphosphate) T: saline laxative P: acid salt	Enemeez Enema*, Fleet Enema*, Fleet Phospho-Soda, Garamycin Ophthalmic Solution*, Saf-Tip Enemas*

T Therapeutic classification.   P Pharmacologic classification.

GENERIC NAME AND CLASSIFICATIONS	TRADE NAMES
sodium polystyrene sulfonate T: potassium-removing resin P: cation-exchange resin	Kayexalate, Resonium A, SPS
sodium salicylate T: nonnarcotic analgesic, antipyretic, anti-inflammatory P: salicylate	Apcogesic*, Bricolide*, Bisalate*, Copavin Compound*, Corilin*, Gaysal-S*, Salcoce*, Uracel-5
sodium thiosalicylate T: nonnarcotic analgesic, antipyretic, anti-inflammatory P: salicylate	Asproject, Rexolate, Tusal
somatrem T: human growth hormone P: anterior pituitary hormone	Protropin
spectinomycin hydrochloride T: antibiotic P: aminocyclitol antibiotic	Trobicin
spironolactone T: management of edema; antihypertensive; diagnosis of primary hyperaldosteronism; treatment of diuretic-induced hypokalemia P: potassium-sparing diuretic	Aldactazide*, Aldactone, Novospiroton†, Sincomen†, Spirotone‡
stanozolol T: angioedema prophylactic P: anabolic steroid	Winstrol
streptokinase T: thrombolytic enzyme P: plasminogen activator	Kabikinase, Streptase
streptomycin sulfate T: antibiotic P: aminoglycoside	Streptomycin Sulfate
streptozocin T: antineoplastic P: alkylating agent, nitrosourea (cell cycle–phase nonspecific)	Zanosar
succimer T: chelating agent P: heavy metal	Chemet

† Available in Canada only.　　‡ Available in Australia only.　　* Combination product.

GENERIC NAME AND CLASSIFICATIONS	TRADE NAMES
succinylcholine chloride (suxamethonium chloride) T: skeletal muscle relaxant P: depolarizing neuromuscular blocking agent	Anectine, Anectine Flo-Pack, Quelicin, Scoline‡, Sucostrin
sucralfate T: antiulcer agent P: pepsin inhibitor	Carafate, Sulcrate†
sufentanil citrate T: analgesic, adjunct to anesthesia, anesthetic P: opioid	Sufenta
sulconazole nitrate T: antifungal agent P: imidazole derivative	Exelderm
sulfacetamide sodium 10% T: antibiotic P: sulfonamide	Acet-Dia-Mer-Sulfonamides*, AK-Sulf Forte, AK-Sulf Ointment, Blephamide Liquifilm*, Blephamide S.O.P.*, Bleph-10 Liquifilm Ophthalmic, Cetamide Ophthalmic, Cetapred Ophthalmic Ointment*, Chero-Trisulfa-V*, Metimyd*, Optimyd*, Sodium Sulamyd 10% Ophthalmic, Sulf-10 Ophthalmic, Vasocidin*
sulfacetamide sodium 15% T: antibiotic P: sulfonamide	Isopto Cetamide Ophthalmic, Sulfacel-15 Ophthalmic, Sulfair 15
sulfacetamide sodium 30% T: antibiotic P: sulfonamide	Sodium Sulamyd 30% Ophthalmic
sulfacytine T: antibiotic P: sulfonamide	Renoquid
sulfadiazine T: antibiotic P: sulfonamide	Acet-Dia-Mer-Sulfonamides*, Chemozine*, Cherasulfa*, Chero-Trisulfa-V*, Lantrisul*, Microsulfon, Silvadene*, Sulfajen Cream*, Triple Sulfa Tab*
sulfamerazine T: antibiotic P: sulfonamide combination	Acet-Dia-Mer-Sulfonamides*, Chemozine*, Cherasulfa*, Chero-Trisulfa-V*, Lantrisul*, Sulfajen Cream*, Triple Sulfa*

GENERIC NAME AND CLASSIFICATIONS

TRADE NAMES

sulfamethazine
T: antibiotic
P: sulfonamide combination

Chemozine*, Cherasulfa*, Lantrisul*, Neotrizine, Sulfajen Cream*, Triple Sulfa*

sulfamethoxazole (sulphamethoxazole)
T: antibiotic
P: sulfonamide

Apo-Sulfamethoxazole†, Azo-Gantanol*, Azo-Gantrisin*, Azosulfisoxazole*, Gantanol, Gantanol DS

sulfasalazine (salazosulfapyridine; sulphasalazine)
T: antibiotic
P: sulfonamide

Azulfidine, Azulfidine EN-Tabs, PMS Sulfasalazine E.C.†, Salazopyrin†‡, Salazopyrin EN-Tabs†‡, S.A.S., S.A.S.-Enteric

sulfinpyrazone
T: renal tubular-blocking agent, platelet aggregation inhibitor
P: uricosuric agent

Anturan†, Anturane

sulfisoxazole (sulfafurazole; sulphafurazole)
T: antibiotic
P: sulfonamide

Azo-Gantrisin*, Azo-Soxazole*, Azo-Sulfisoxazole†‡, Azo-Sulfizin*, Azo-Urizole*, Gantrisin, Lipo Gantrisin, Novosoxazole†, Rosoxol-Azo*, Vagilia Cream*, Velmatrol-A*

sulindac
T: nonnarcotic analgesic, antipyretic, anti-inflammatory
P: nonsteroidal anti-inflammatory

Clinoril

T

tamoxifen citrate
T: antineoplastic
P: nonsteroidal antiestrogen

Nolvadex, Nolvadex D†‡, Tamofen†

temazepam
T: sedative-hypnotic
P: benzodiazepine

Restoril, Temaz

teniposide (VM-26)
T: antineoplastic
P: podophyllotoxin (cell cycle-phase specific, G_2 and late S phases)

Vumon‡

terazosin hydrochloride
T: antihypertensive
P: selective $alpha_1$ blocker

Hytrin

terbutaline sulfate
T: bronchodilator, tocolytic
P: adrenergic ($beta_2$ agonist)

Brethaire, Brethine, Bricanyl

terconazole
T: antifungal
P: triazole derivative

Terazol 3 Vaginal Suppositories, Terazol 7 Vaginal Cream

terfenadine
T: antihistamine (H_1-receptor antagonist)
P: butyrophenone derivative

Seldane, Teldane‡

terpin hydrate
T: expectorant
P: aliphatic alcohol

Anti-Tussive*, Chexit*, Glynaphen*, Tussagesic*, Tussaminic*

testolactone
T: antineoplastic
P: androgen

Teslac

testosterone
T: androgen replacement, antineoplastic
P: androgen

Andeone*, Andesterone*, Andro, Android-G*, Andronaq, Anestro*, Angen*, Depo-Testadiol*, Di-Hormone*, Di-Met*, Diorpin*, Di-Steroid*, Estratest*, Estrone-Testosterone Vial*, Geramine*, Geratic Forte*, Geriamic*, Geritag*, Histerone, Horm-Triad*, Malogen*, Tesogen*, Testaqua,

---

GENERIC NAME AND CLASSIFICATIONS	TRADE NAMES
testosterone *(continued)*	Testrone*, Testoject, Tripole-F*, Vi-Testrogen*
testosterone cypionate T: androgen replacement, antineoplastic P: androgen	Andro-Cyp, Andronaq-LA, Andronate, D-Diol*, dep Andro, Depotest, Depo-Testadiol*, Depotestogen*, Depo-Testosterone, Dep-Testradiol*, Duratest, Duo-Cyp*, Duracrine*, Estram-C*, Span F.M.*, T-Cypionate, T.E. Lonate*, Tesionate, Testa-C, Testoject-LA, Testred Cypionate, Virilon IM
testosterone enanthate T: androgen replacement, antineoplastic P: androgen	Android-T, Andro-LA, Andryl, Ardiol*, Deladumone*, Delatestadiol*, Delatestryl, Ditate DS*, Duoval-P.A.*, Durathate, Everone, Malogex†, Repose-TE*, Retadiamone*, Span-Est-Test*, Teev Preps*, Testanate #2 & 3*, Testone LA, Testrin PA, Valertest*
testosterone propionate T: androgen replacement, antineoplastic P: androgen	Malogen†, Testex
tetanus antitoxin (TAT), equine T: tetanus antitoxin P: antitoxin	
tetanus immune globulin, human T: tetanus prophylaxis agent P: immune serum	Homo-Tet, Hu-Tet, Hyper-Tet†
tetanus toxoid, adsorbed; tetanus toxoid, fluid T: tetanus prophylaxis agent P: toxoid	
tetracaine T: ophthalmic local anesthetic P: ester-type local anesthetic	Pontocaine Eye
tetracaine hydrochloride T: local anesthetic, topical anesthetic, spinal anesthetic P: ester-type anesthetic	Cetacaine*, Isotraine*, Pontocaine

GENERIC NAME AND CLASSIFICATIONS	TRADE NAMES
tetracycline T: antibiotic P: tetracycline	Achryomycin Ophthalmic, Mysteclin*
tetracycline hydrochloride T: antibiotic P: tetracycline	Achromycin, Achromycin V*, Apo-Tetra†, Austramycin V‡, Bristacycline, Comycin*, Cyclopar, Hostacycline P‡, Kesso-Tetra, Nor-Tet, Novotetra†, Panmycin, Panmycin P‡, Robitet, Sarocycline, Sumycin, Tetracap, Tetracyn, Tetralan, Tetralean†, Topicycline
tetrahydrozoline hydrochloride T: vasoconstrictor, decongestant P: sympathomimetic agent	Murine Plus, Optigene, Soothe, Tetrasine, Tyzine Drops, Tyzine Pediatric Drops, Visine
theophylline T: bronchodilator P: xanthine derivative	*Immediate-release liquids:* Accurbron, Aerolate, Aquaphyllin, Asmalix, Broncotabs*, Bronkaid*, Bronkodyl, Bronkodyl S-R, Bronkolixir*, Co-Xan*, Duraphyl, Elixicon, Elixomin, Elixophyllin, Elixophyllin-KI*, Elixophyllin SR, Eponal*, Iso-Asminyl*, Isophed*, Lanophyllin, Lardet*, Lixolin, Lodrane, Marax DF Syrup*, Marax Tabs*, Medihaler-Iso*, Neogen*, Nuelin‡, Nuelin-SR‡, Panaphyllin*, Quibron*, Quibron-300*, Quibron Plus*, Quibron-T/SR, Respbid, Slo-Bid Gyrocaps, Slo-Phyllin, Slo-Phyllin GG*, Somophyllin-CRT*, Somophyllin-T *Immediate-release tablets and capsules:* Bronkodyl, Theophyl-SR, Theospan SR, Theo-Time, Theovent Long-acting, Uniphyl *Timed-release capsules:* Aerolate *Timed-release tablets:* Constant-T, Sustaire, Synophylate GG*, Tedral Elixir*, Tedral SA*, Theobid Duracaps, Theobid Jr., Theochron, Theocolate*, Theo-Dur, Theo-Dur Sprinkles, Theolair, Theolair-SR, Theon, Theophyl, Theo-24
theophylline sodium glycinate T: bronchodilator P: xanthine derivative	Acet-Am†, Asbron G*, Synophedal*, Synophylate, Synophylate-GG*, Synophylate with Phenobarbital*, TSG Croup Liquid*, TSG-KI*

T Therapeutic classification.   P Pharmacologic classification.

GENERIC NAME AND CLASSIFICATIONS	TRADE NAMES
thiabendazole T: anthelmintic P: benzimidazole	Mintezol
thiethylperazine maleate T: antiemetic P: phenothiazine derivative	Norzine, Torecan
thioguanine (6-thioguan-ine; 6-TG) T: antineoplastic P: antimetabolite (cell cycle–phase specific, S phase)	Lanvis†
thiopental sodium (thiopen-tone sodium) T: intravenous anesthetic P: barbiturate	Intraval Sodium‡, Pentothal Sodium
thioridazine hydrochloride T: antipsychotic P: phenothiazine (piperidine derivative)	Aldazine‡, Apo-Thioridazine†, Mellaril, Mellaril-S, Novoridazine†, PMS Thioridazine†
thiotepa T: antineoplastic P: alkylating agent (cell cycle–phase nonspecific)	Thiotepa
thiothixene T: antipsychotic P: thioxanthene	Navane
thiothixene hydrochloride T: antipsychotic P: thioxanthene	Navane
thrombin T: topical hemostatic P: enzyme	Thrombinar, Thrombostat‡
thyroglobulin T: thyroid agent P: thyroid hormone	Proloid
thyroid dessicated T: thyroid agent P: thyroid hormone	Armour Thyroid, S-P-T, Thyrar, Thyroid Strong, Thyroid USP Enseals, Thyro-Teric
thyrotropin (thyroid-stimu-lating hormone or TSH) T: thyrotropic hormone P: anterior pituitary hormone	Thytropar

† Available in Canada only.   ‡ Available in Australia only.   * Combination product.

GENERIC NAME AND CLASSIFICATIONS	TRADE NAMES
ticarcillin disodium T: antibiotic P: extended-spectrum penicillin, alpha-carboxypenicillin	Ticar, Ticillin‡
ticarcillin disodium/ clavulanate potassium T: antibiotic P: extended-spectrum penicillin, beta-lactamase inhibitor	Timentin
ticlodipine T: stroke preventative P: platelet inhibitor	Ticlid
timolol maleate T: antihypertensive agent, adjunct in myocardial infarction, antiglaucoma agent P: beta-adrenergic blocking agent	Apo-Timol†, Blocadren, MITimoptic Solution, Timolide*
tioconazole T: antifungal P: imidazole derivative	Vagistat
tiopronin T: cystine-solubilizing agent P: thiol compound	Thiola
tobramycin T: antibiotic P: aminoglycoside	Tobrex
tobramycin sulfate T: antibiotic P: aminoglycoside	Nebcin
tocainide hydrochloride T: ventricular antiarrhythmic P: local anesthetic (amide type)	Tonocard
tolazamide T: antidiabetic agent P: sulfonylurea	Ronase, Tolamide, Tolinase
tolazoline hydrochloride T: antihypertensive P: peripheral vasodilator, alpha-adrenergic blocking agent	Priscoline

T Therapeutic classification.   P Pharmacologic classification.

GENERIC NAME AND CLASSIFICATIONS	TRADE NAMES
tolbutamide T: antidiabetic agent P: sulfonylurea	Apo-Tolbutamide†, Mobenol†, Novobutamide†, Oramide, Orinase
tolmetin sodium T: nonnarcotic analgesic, antipyretic, anti-inflammatory P: nonsteroidal anti-inflammatory	Tolectin, Tolectin DS
tolnaftate T: topical antifungal agent P: synthetic antifungal agent	Aftate for Athlete's Foot, Aftate for Jock Itch, Footwork, Fungatin, Genaspor, NP-27, Tinactin, Zeasorb-AF
tolrestat T: treatment of diabetic complications P: carboxylic acid (aldose reductase inhibitor)	Alderase
tranylcypromine sulfate T: antidepressant P: monoamine oxidase inhibitor	Parnate
trazodone hydrochloride T: antidepressant P: triazolopyridine derivative	Desyrel, Trazon, Trialodine
tretinoin (vitamin A acid; retinoic acid) T: antiacne agent P: vitamin A derivative	Retin-A, StieVAA†
triamcinolone T: anti-inflammatory, immunosuppressant P: glucocorticoid	Aristocort, Atolone, Kenacort, Mycolog*, Tricilone
triamcinolone acetonide T: anti-inflammatory, immunosuppressant P: glucocorticoid	Cenocort A, Cinonide, Kenaject, Kenalog, Kenalone‡, Mycolog*, Tac-3, Tramacort, Triam-A, Triamonide, Tri-Kort, Trilog
triamcinolone acetonide (topical) T: topical anti-inflammatory P: glucocorticoid	Aristocort, Kenalog, Kenalone‡
triamcinolone diacetate T: anti-inflammatory, immunosuppressant P: glucocorticoid	Amcort, Aristocort Forte, Aristocort Intralesional, Articulose-L.A., Cenocort Forte, Cinalone, Kenacort, Triam-Forte, Trilone, Tristoject

† Available in Canada only.   ‡ Available in Australia only.   * Combination product.

GENERIC NAME AND CLASSIFICATIONS	TRADE NAMES
triamcinolone hexacetonide T: anti-inflammatory, immunosuppressant P: injectable glucocorticoid	Aristospan Intra-articular, Aristospan Intralesional
triamterene T: diuretic P: potassium-sparing diuretic	Dyazide*, Dyrenium, Dytac‡
triazolam T: sedative-hypnotic P: benzodiazepine	Halcion
trichlormethiazide T: diuretic, antihypertensive P: thiazide diuretic	Aquazide, Diurese, Metahydrin, Metatensin*, Naqua, Naquival*
trientine hydrochloride T: heavy metal antagonist P: chelating agent	Cuprid
triethanolamine polypeptide oleate-condensate T: cerumenolytic P: oleic acid derivative	Cerumenex
trifluoperazine hydrochloride T: antipsychotic, antiemetic P: phenothiazine (piperazine derivative)	Apo-Trifluoperazine†, Calmazine‡, Novo-Flurazine†, Solazine†, Stelazine, Suprazine, Terfluzine†
trifluridine T: antiviral agent P: fluorinated pyrimidine nucleoside	Viroptic Ophthalmic Solution 1%
trihexyphenidyl hydrochloride T: antiparkinsonian agent P: anticholinergic	Aparkane†, Apo-Trihex†, Artane, Artane Sequels, Novohexidyl†, Trihexane, Trihexy-2, Trihexy-5
trilostane T: adrenocortical suppressant P: synthetic steroid	Modrastane
trimebutine maleate T: antispasmotic P: unclassified	Modulon†
trimeprazine tartrate T: antipruritic P: phenothiazine-derivative antihistamine	Panectyl†, Temaril

---

T Therapeutic classification.   P Pharmacologic classification.

GENERIC NAME AND CLASSIFICATIONS	TRADE NAMES
trimethadione T: anticonvulsant P: oxazolidinedione derivative	Tridione
trimethaphan camsylate T: antihypertensive P: ganglionic blocking agent	Arfonad
trimethobenzamide hydrochloride T: antiemetic P: ethanolamine-related antihistamine	Tebamide, Tegamide, Ticon, Tigan, Tiject-20
trimethoprim T: antibiotic P: synthetic folate antagonist	Alprin‡, Bactrim*, Proloprim, Septra*, Septra DS*, Trimpex, Triprim‡
trimetrexate gluconate T: antimicrobial, antineoplastic P: dihydrofolate reductase inhibitor	
trimipramine maleate T: antidepressant, antianxiety agent P: tricyclic antidepressant	Apo-Trimip†, Surmontil
tripelennamine citrate T: antihistamine (H_1-receptor antagonist) P: ethylenediamine-derivative antihistamine	PBZ
tripelennamine hydrochloride T: antihistamine (H_1-receptor antagonist) P: alkylamine antihistamine derivative	Actifed*, Actifed-C Syrup*, Atridine*, PBZ, PBZ-SR, Pelamine, Pyribenzamine
triprolidine hydrochloride T: antihistamine (H_1-receptor antagonist) P: alkylamine antihistamine derivative	Actidil, Myidyl
tromethamine T: systemic alkalinizer P: sodium-free organic amine	Tham

---

† Available in Canada only.   ‡ Available in Australia only.   * Combination product.

GENERIC NAME AND CLASSIFICATIONS	TRADE NAMES
tropicamide T: cycloplegic, mydriatic P: anticholinergic agent	Mydriacyl, Tropicacyl
tuberculin purified protein derivative (PPD) T: diagnostic skin test antigen P: *Mycobacterium tuberculosis* and *Mycobacterium bovis* antigen	Aplisol, PPD-stabilized Solution (Mantoux test), Tubersol
tuberculosis multiple-puncture tests T: diagnostic skin test antigen P: *Mycobacterium tuberculosis* and *Mycobacterium bovis* antigen	Aplitest (dried purified protein derivative [PPD]), Mono-Vacc Test (liquid Old Tuberculin [OT]), Sclavo Test (dried PPD), Tine Test (dried OT; dried PPD)
tubocurarine chloride T: skeletal muscle relaxant P: nondepolarizing neuromuscular blocking agent	Tubarine†
typhoid vaccine T: bacterial vaccine P: vaccine	

UV

GENERIC NAME AND CLASSIFICATIONS	TRADE NAMES
undecylenic acid and zinc undecylenate T: topical antifungal P: undecylenate salt	Cruex, Desenex, Desenex Aerosol, Quinsana Plus, Ting Spray, Tulvex*
uracil mustard T: antineoplastic P: alkylating agent (cell cycle–phase nonspecific)	Uracil Mustard Capsules
urea (carbamide) T: osmotic diuretic P: carbonic acid salt	Akne Drying Lotion*, Carmol-HC Cream*, Kerid Ear Drops*, Teenac*, 20-Cain Burn Relief*, Ureaphil
urokinase T: thrombolytic enzyme P: thrombolytic enzyme	Abbokinase, Ukidan‡, Win-Kinase
ursodiol T: gallstone solubilizing agent P: bile acid	Actigall
valproate sodium T: anticonvulsant P: carboxylic acid derivative	Depakene Syrup, Epilim‡, Myproic Acid Syrup
valproic acid T: anticonvulsant P: carboxylic acid derivative	Dalpro, Depa, Depakene, Myproic Acid
vancomycin hydrochloride T: antibiotic P: glycopeptide	Vancocin
varicella-zoster immune globulin (VZIG) T: varicella-zoster prophy-laxis agent P: immune serum	
vasopressin (antidiuretic hormone) T: antidiuretic hormone, peri-staltic stimulant, hemostatic agent P: posterior pituitary hormone	Pitressin

---

† Available in Canada only.   ‡ Available in Australia only.   * Combination product.

GENERIC NAME AND CLASSIFICATIONS	TRADE NAMES
vasopressin tannate T: treatment of diabetes insipidus, post-operative distention, diagnostic aid P: polypeptide hormone	Pitressin Tannate
vecuronium bromide T: skeletal muscle relaxant P: nondepolarizing neuromuscular blocking agent	Norcuron
verapamil hydrochloride T: antianginal, antihypertensive, antiarrhythmic P: calcium channel blocker	Calan, Calan SR, Cordilox Oral‡, Isoptin, Isoptin SR, Veradil‡
vidarabine T: antiviral agent P: purine nucleoside	Vira-A Ophthalmic
vidarabine monohydrate (adenine arabinoside; ara-A) T: antiviral agent P: purine nucleoside	Vira-A
vinblastine sulfate (VLB) T: antineoplastic P: vinca alkaloid (cell cycle–phase specific, M phase)	Alkaban-AQ, Velban, Velbe†‡, Velsar
vincristine sulfate T: antineoplastic P: vinca alkaloid (cell cycle–phase specific, M phase)	Oncovin, Vincasar PFS
vindesine sulfate T: antineoplastic P: vinca alkaloid (cell cycle–phase specific, M phase)	Eldisine†
vitamin A (retinol) T: vitamin P: fat-soluble vitamin	Acon, Aquasol A, Tri-Vi-Flor*, Vicon Forte*, Vicon Plus*, Vi-Zac*
vitamin B₁ (thiamine hydrochloride) T: vitamin supplement P: B-complex vitamin	Albee with Vitamin C*, Apatate Drops, Betalin S, Betamin‡, Beta-Sol‡, Biamine, Cenalene*, Nycralan*, Thia, Z-Bec

---

T Therapeutic classification.   P Pharmacologic classification.

GENERIC NAME AND CLASSIFICATIONS	TRADE NAMES
vitamin B₂ (riboflavin) T: vitamin supplement P: B-complex vitamin	Albee with Vitamin C*, Riboflavin with Niacinamide*, Vicon Forte*, Z-Bec*
vitamin B₃ (niacin, nicotinic acid) T: vitamin supplement, antilipemic, peripheral vasodilator P: B-complex vitamin	Albee with Vitamins*, Lipo-Nicin*, Myodyne*, Niac, Nialexo-C*, Nico-400, Nicobid, Nicolar, Ni-Span, Z-Bec*
vitamin B₃ (niacinamide, nicotinamide) T: vitamin supplement P: B-complex vitamin	Cenalene*, Iodo-Niacin*, Lipo-Nicin*, Pergrava #2*, P.S.P. IV Injectable*, Riboflavin and Niacinamide*, Rite-Diet*, Solu-Pred*, Vicon-C*, Vicon Forte*, Vicon Plus*, Vi-Testrogen*
vitamin B₆ (pyridoxine hydrochloride) T: nutritional supplement P: B-complex vitamin	Albee with Vitamin C*, Beesix, Calpas Isozine*, Calpas-INAH-6*, Hexa-Betalin, Hexacrest, Nestrex, Niadox*, Pasna Tri-Pack*, P-I-N Forte*, Teebaconin*, Triniad Plus 30*, Uniad Plus*, Vicon Forte*, Z-Bec*
vitamin B₉ (folic acid) T: vitamin supplement P: folic acid derivative	C-Ron F.A.*, Fero-Folic-500*, Folvite, Folvron*, Intrin*, Novofolacid†, Pergrava #2*
vitamin B₁₂ (cyanocobalamin) T: vitamin, nutrition supplement P: water-soluble vitamin	Anacobin†, Bedoce, Bedoz†, Betalin 12, Bioglan B₁₂ Plus‡, Cenalene*, Crystamine, Cyanabin†, Cyanocobalamin, Cyano-Gel, Dodex, Intrin*, Kaybovite, Poyamin, Redisol, Rubesol-1000, Rubion†, Rubramin, Sigamine, Stuart Amino Acids and B₁₂*, Vicon Forte*, Z-Bec
vitamin B₁₂ₐ (hydroxocobalamin) T: vitamin, nutrition supplement P: water-soluble vitamin	Alpha-Ruvite, Codroxomin, Droxomin, Rubesol-L.A.
vitamin C (ascorbic acid) T: vitamin P: water-soluble vitamin	Aerolone Compound*, Albee with Vitamin C*, Ascorbicap, Bisalate*, Cebid Timecelles, Centuss*, Cetane, Cevalin, Cevi-Bid, Ce-Vi-Sol, Cevita, Chew-Hist*, C-Ron*, C-Span, Cytoferin*, Dull-C, Eldofe-C*, Ferancee*, Ferancee HP*, Fero-Folic-500*, Fero-Grad-500*, Ferropyl Chew- *(continued)*

GENERIC NAME AND CLASSIFICATIONS	TRADE NAMES
vitamin C *(continued)*	Tab*, Flavettes‡, Gaysal-S*, Hemaspan*, Hescor-K*, I.L.X. with Vitamin B_{12}*, Intrin*, Mol-Iron with Vitamin C*, Nialexo-C*, Recoup*, Redoxon†, Rependo*, Rinocidin*, Solucap C, Stuart Hematinic*, Tri-Vi-Flor*, Vicon-C*, Vicon Forte*, Vicon Plus*, Vita C Crystals, Vi-Zac*, Z-Bec*
vitamin D T: vitamin P: fat-soluble vitamin	Elekap*, Tri-Vi-Flor*
vitamin D_2 (ergocalciferol) T: vitamin P: fat-soluble vitamin	Calciferol, Drisdol, Radiostol†, Radiostol Forte‡, Vitamin D
vitamin D_3 (cholecalciferol) T: vitamin P: fat-soluble vitamin	Delta-D, Vitamin D_3
vitamin K_1 (phytonadione) T: treatment of hypothrom-binemia caused by vitamin K deficiency P: naphthoquinone derivative	AquaMEPHYTON, Konakion, Mephyton
vitamin K_3 (menadione-menadiol soldium diphosphate) T: blood coagulation modifier P: vitamin K	C.V.P. with Vitamins*, Hescor-K*, Redendo*, Synkavite†, Synkayvite

T Therapeutic classification.   P Pharmacologic classification.

WXYZ

GENERIC NAME AND CLASSIFICATIONS	TRADE NAMES
warfarin sodium T: anticoagulant P: coumadin derivative	Coumadin, Panwarfin, Warfilone Sodium†
xylometazoline hydrochloride T: decongestant, vasoconstrictor P: sympathomimetic	4-Way Long Acting, Neo-Synephrine II, Otrivin, Sine-Off Nasal Spray, Sinex-L.A.
yellow fever vaccine T: viral vaccine P: vaccine	YF-Vax
zidovudine (azidothymidine; AZT) T: antiviral P: thymidine analog	Retrovir
zinc oxide T: nutritional supplement, topical anti-infective P: trace element	Acne Drying Lotion*, Anocaine*, Anugesic*, Anulan*, Anusol*, Anusol HC*, Biscolan*, Biscolan HC*, Derma Medi-Cone-HC*, Doctient HC*, Pazo*, Pile-Gon*, Rectacort*, Unguentine Plus*, Wyanoids*, Wyanoids HC*, Xylocaine Suppositories*, Ziradryl*
zinc sulfate T: nutritional supplement, topical anti-infective P: trace element	Acnederm Lotion*, Bromidrosis Crystals*, Bufopto Zinc Sulfate, Eye-Sed Ophthalmic, Mass pH Powder*, M-Z Drops*, Op-Thal-Zin, Phenylzin*, Prefrin-Z*, Vicon-C*, Vicon Forte*, Vicon Plus*, Z-Bec*, Zinc-220*

Index

B

C

D

E

H

I

JK

P

Phyllocontin, 7
Physeptone, 83
phytonadione, 138
Pile-Gon, 17, 139
Pilocar, 106
Pilocarpine, 48
Pilocel, 106
Pilofrin Liquifilm, 106
Pilomiotin, 106
Pilopine HS, 106
Pilopt, 106
Pima, 109
Pindac, 106
Pinex Regular, 109
Pin-Tega Tabs, 107
piperadine derivative, 77
piperazine, 107
    derivative antihistamine, 18, 34, 81
    estrone sulfate, 51
piperidine antihistamine, 12
    derivative, 35
piperidine central nervous system stim-
    ulant, 86
piperidine dione, 59
    derivative, 86
piperonyl butoxide and petroleum dis-
    tillate combination, 114
Pipracil, 107
Pipril, 107
Piriton, 28, 98
Pitressin, 135
Pitressin Tannate, 136
Placidyl, 51
Plaquenil, 67
Plasbumin 5%, 4
Plasbumin 25%, 4
Plasmanate, 107
Plasma-Plex, 107
Plasmatein, 107
plasma volume expander, 4, 38, 64,
    107
    blood derivative, 4
plasminogen activator, 123
Platamine, 30
platelet
    aggregation inhibitor, 43, 125
    inhibitor, 130
Platinol, 30

Plegine, 102
Plendil, 54
Plexonal, 42, 103, 121
P-I-N Forte, 73, 137
PMB 200, 82
P.M.P., 104
P.M.P. Expectorant, 28, 32, 61
PMS Benztropine, 15
PMS-Dimenhydrinate, 42
PMS-Isoniazid, 73
PMS Metronidazole, 87
PMS Nylidrin, 95
PMS Procyclidine, 112
PMS-Promethazine, 112
PMS-Propranolol, 113
PMS Pyrazinamide, 114
PMS Sulfasalazine E.C., 125
PMS Thioridazine, 129
Pneumovax 23, 107
Pnu-Imune 23, 107
podophyllotoxin, 53, 125
Point-Two, 122
Poladex TD, 38
Polaramine, 38
Polaramine Expectorant, 38, 61
Polaramine Repetabs, 38
Polargen, 38
Polarmine Expectorant, 114
polyanhydroglucuronic acid, 97
Polycillin, 9
Polycillin-N, 8
Polycillin-PRB, 8, 111
Polyectin, 32, 61, 72, 104, 105
polyene macrolide, 8, 95
    antibiotic, 92
Polymox, 8
polysaccharide, synthetic, 38
Polysporin, 13, 108
Polysporin Spray, 13
Polytuss-DM, 28, 39, 61
polyvinyl alcohol or cellulose, deriva-
    tives of, 10
Ponderal, 54
Ponderal Pacaps, 54
Ponderax, 54
Ponderax Pacaps, 54
Pondimin, 54
Pondimin Extentabs, 54

W